Contents

Acknowledgments

I wish to thank my colleagues and staff members who encouraged me in pursuing this project. I'd like especially to thank those who, in their busy schedules, provided invaluable help to me in writing this book: Julie Berry for showing me the concept of the book; Christine Lee, my senior staff member; and patient coordinator Elena Molina. I also thank Julie Hoff, R.N., of the Gold Coast Med Spa, whose knowledge is synergistic to my patients' care. I thank Laura Wallace, who served as editor for this book, for her inestimable help in bringing the book to life. Finally, I extend my thanks to Susan Adams, managing editor at Addicus Books, for her work in the final stages of editing.

Michael Byun, M.D.

I would like to thank my wonderful family for all of the support and love they share with me. I am especially grateful to have recognized the value of life and the courage to survive that my father has provided me. Of course, the love and magic of living is valued every day as I embrace the life and the joy that Hanny and Benny bring to me every day.

I would also like to extend my sincere thanks and gratitude to my outstanding family of associates that I have been fortunate enough to work with daily. Their dedication to our vision and our patients are second to none. Their tireless efforts are recognized and greatly appreciated. Thank You.

I would also like to thank all of the patients to whom I have been fortunate enough to meet. Every day I receive tremendous satisfaction in knowing that the relationships I have developed with you will last a lifetime. I enjoy educating and being educated by you, and hope that I can continue to provide care to you for years to come.

Finally, my wife, Hope. Thank you for your patience, support and loving devotion. Thank you also for your unselfishness which is demonstrated every day by your exceptional love and care for Hanny and Benny.

Jon Mendelsohn, M.D.

I would like to thank those who helped make it possible for me to participate in this book project. I thank my wife, Lynn Malcolm Truswell, J.D, who is my practice manager, my attorney, and my friend. I am particularly blessed with a marvelous office staff who make my day-to-day life run smoothly and enjoyably.

My clinical staff—Laura Tasker, Kathy Rollet, Lisa Cowan, and Cozette Brodeur—guide the patients through the cosmetic surgery process with kindness and compassion. My skin-care technicians/make-up artists, Johanne Barron and Katina Haslam, are experts on chemical peels and microdermabrasion and add the final touch of cosmetics to the work I do.

My front office staff, Nancy Edgington and Darci Cintron, are the best where first impressions count. I also thank Margaret Ancira of Physician's Choice Arizona and David Reike, Vice President of Marketing, Atrium Medical Corporation, for their contributions. My praise goes to our editor, Laura Wallace, whose editorial guidance helped make this book a reality. Finally, I acknowledge the American Academy of Facial Plastic and Reconstructive Surgery, the organization that guides, nurtures, and educates the experts in my specialty.

William H. Truswell, M.D.

Introduction

One of our society's most striking features is that we are healthier and more vigorous than ever before. The passing years? Forget about them. We're just as young as our dreams.

Brave words, and we believe them. At the same time, we all know we're living in a youth culture. It's part Hollywood, part Madison Avenue. It's not just vanity that makes us want to look our energetic best, however. There are also real frustrations.

Ageism exists in the workplace, whether we like it or not. Even with a wealth of well-earned savvy, you may feel disadvantaged on the job. Likewise, it can be harder to enjoy a vibrant sexuality when the media blares that it belongs only to the young.

The good news? Today, there's a tremendous amount you can do to restore and rejuvenate your appearance so that the way you look is much more in tune with the way you think and feel. And you might be surprised at how non-drastic many of the latest methods are.

The focus of this book is on the newest facial rejuvenation techniques that require no invasive surgery. Changes ranging from subtle to amazing are made possible through cutting-edge technologies that forgo the "cutting edge" completely. Other procedures require only single incisions so tiny that they leave no scars. Recovery is easier, too. Many of these new procedures result in remarkable transformations with a minimum of inconvenience or downtime. Some can literally be done on a lunch hour.

Here, you'll find a comprehensive look at the latest non-invasive treatments and learn how you, too, can have a "nonsurgical facelift."

One

Your Skin & Facial Rejuvenation

Your Skin & Facial Rejuvenation

Whatever age you are now, you may have already noticed some of the signs of aging in your mirror. The degrees and types of changes vary from person to person, of course, but aging is a universal experience. No one is immune from it.

Almost all of us appear fresh-faced throughout our twenties. Only in the late twenties do we begin to notice fine lines and more persistent freckles, the forerunners of age spots. In our thirties, we may see a few more stubborn patches of uneven pigmentation. We may notice early wrinkling—smile lines that linger or a frown line that shows most of the time. Skin tone may be changing too, with areas that appear thinner, thicker, or rougher than they used to be.

In our forties, gravity seems to play a role in the aging process. The skin loses some of its elasticity and a bit of sagging may appear, perhaps along the jawline or under the eyes. Unwanted hairs may begin to sprout along the chin and lip as hormone levels fluctuate. New wrinkles are more pronounced.

In our fifties and beyond, these changes increase. Deeper lines and wrinkles appear. In facial folds or wrinkles, the skin's thickness can shrink to just one third of that of the surrounding skin. Other changes may include the appearance of age spots and spider veins.

Still, there's no need to be disheartened. Instead, now you can explore a constellation of remarkable nonsurgical treatments that will allow you to have much smoother, more luminous, firmer, and younger-looking skin—no matter what decade you're in.

Anatomy of Skin

The skin is an amazing organ. Yes, it *is* considered an organ. In fact, it's the body's largest organ, weighing about six pounds. The skin takes care of us in ways we rarely even think about. It acts as a shield for the entire body, protecting us from heat, injury, and infection. It also regulates body temperature and stores water. And through the sense of touch it delivers the sensations of both pain and pleasure.

The skin is made up of three layers:

- epidermis: the outer layer of the skin

- dermis: the middle layer

- subcutis: the deepest layer

The *epidermis* actually has several layers itself, and as the cells move up through these layers, they form the tougher outer surface of our skin. By the time they reach the surface, the cells are actually dead and they flake off.

The *dermis* layer contains blood vessels, lymph vessels, hair follicles, and sweat glands. These elements are held together by connective tissues, including *collagen* and *elastin*, which give the skin its strength and elasticity.

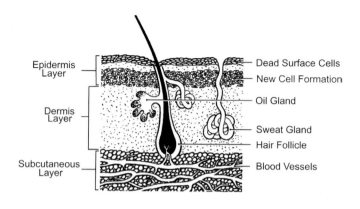

The *subcutis*, or subcutaneous layer, is made up of a network of collagen and fat cells. This deepest layer acts as an insulator, holding in body heat. The fat layer also "fills out" the skin, giving it plumpness.

Why Skin Ages

As we age, the connective tissues in the skin's dermis layer begin to break down and cells start losing their ability to repair themselves. With less collagen and elastin, the skin starts to wrinkle and sag. At the same time, skin is unable to retain as much moisture as it did in younger days, and skin becomes drier and thinner. Drier skin means aging skin. Several factors affect the way our skin ages.

Sun Damage

You may have thought that simply getting older was the reason your face ages. To some degree, certainly, chronological aging leaves its marks on your face. But the truth is that the single most powerful force working to alter your smooth, healthy skin is sun exposure. Sun causes *photoaging* or premature wrinkling. From sunburns and tanning to the cumulative effects of brief daily exposure such as going out to the mailbox, exposure to the sun is the biggest cause of an aged appearance. It's estimated that 80 percent of aging of the skin is caused by the sun. And the greater portion of that sun damage has occurred by the time you are twenty years old.

Just as the ultraviolet rays in sunlight can fade fabrics and erode the finish on your car, they also wreak havoc on your skin. Two types of ultraviolet (UV) rays do the damage. *UV-A* rays gradually and invisibly weaken collagen, the protein-rich supporting layer that keeps your skin firm, supple, and wrinkle-resistant. *UV-B* rays cause burning and tanning and set

the stage for skin cancer. Tanning beds or lamps are no exception—they also damage your skin.

Tanning may create the appearance of being healthy, but its effect on the skin is anything but healthy. Tanning is actually the skin's way of trying to protect itself from the sun. Sure, a tan may look good, but that short-term glow has very unpleasant long-term consequences.

Here's a simple way to evaluate your level of sun damage. Compare the skin of your face to the skin of your buttocks, breasts, or inner upper arm. It's no coincidence that the parts of

Ranges of Ultraviolet Rays

- UV-A rays are longer, penetrate more deeply, and are associated with premature aging.

- UV-B rays are shorter, but cause sunburns.

- UV-C rays are filtered by the earth's ozone layer and are not as threatening to skin.

your body that have been well shielded from the sun look and feel so much younger. By every conceivable measure, and no matter what your natural skin tone or ethnicity, we'll say it again—the sun is your skin's biggest enemy.

Today, you're also much more vulnerable to devastating skin cancers than people used to be. Because of the depletion of the earth's ozone layer, far more radiation from the sun reaches you every day. The rate of skin cancer—including the deadliest form, melanoma—has increased by about 30 percent in the last twenty years.

Genes, Gravity, and Unhealthy Habits

Without a doubt, our genetics play a part in our health, including the rate at which our skin ages. To get a glimpse of what your genes suggest, take a look at your family. You may have inherited a tendency to frown, a furrowed brow, or a fair complexion. If you've always been told you look like an older relative, the patterns of aging in that relative's face may reflect what you're beginning to see in your own. It's simply your genetic blueprint.

Simple gravity also has a subtle effect on your face. A natural downward pull encourages facial tissues to sag over time. Likewise, if you've been carrying extra pounds, the excess weight can also tug your face downward, creating a tired, droopy expression. If you've dieted off and on, your skin may have stretched, which also contributes to sagging.

What about unhealthy habits? Skin-sabotaging habits include smoking, drinking, and a poor diet. Smoking decreases the healthy blood flow that brings oxygen and nutrients to your skin, and the constant puckering and squinting cause wrinkles. Anything beyond moderate alcohol consumption on a regular basis dehydrates your skin and produces a pasty, sallow complexion. And a poor diet undermines your skin at every turn—without balanced nutrition your skin cells can't renew themselves at a normal rate. A diet that's short on major nutrients also dims your skin's ability to fight off the effects of environmental pollutants.

Types of Wrinkles

As we age, we experience two basic types of wrinkles: *dynamic wrinkles* and *static wrinkles*. Lines caused by repeated facial expressions are called dynamic wrinkles. In other words, they form because of our actions. On the other hand, wrinkles that stay visible whether or not you're making facial expressions are known as *static* wrinkles. They stay put. How to tell the difference? Relax your face and look in the mirror. Any wrinkles you see are static ones. Now frown, and you'll see a pronounced vertical crease or two; or smile, and crow's feet may form at the corners of your eyes. These are dynamic wrinkles.

What Is Facial Skin Rejuvenation?

The term *facial rejuvenation* refers to treating the skin in such a way as to make it look younger. And today, there is no shortage in the number of treatments. In fact, an explosion has occurred in nonsurgical, or *non-invasive,* cosmetic procedures, those performed on or just under the skin.

Depending on the types of problems you'd like to have corrected, you can choose from a wide array of options. Some of them have been around a while. Others are newer, high-tech techniques. For example, to repair and restore sun-damaged skin, a partial- or full-face chemical peel may do the job. Laser skin resurfacing, done with a computer-driven laser, is another option.

In this book you'll find detailed, comprehensive information on all the most popular facial rejuvenation procedures available today, including:

- *Chemical peels*: topical solutions that remove layers of aged skin

- *Microdermabrasion*: subtle "sanding" for a younger skin surface

- *Wrinkle fillers*: injections and implants for lines and contours

- *Botox*: injections to relax wrinkles

- *Lasers*: beams of light that correct skin defects

- *Lip augmentation*: injections to achieve fuller lips

Many of these procedures require minimal recovery time and can be easily worked into a busy schedule. The short-term aftereffects, such as redness or mild bruising, can usually be camouflaged with makeup. Most people go right back to work, or at most, have the procedure done on a Friday, relax over the weekend, and return to work on Monday.

Still, it is important to remember that just because these procedures are nonsurgical, they are not "non-medical." So rather than heading into the nearest spa that may advertise some of these treatments, it's very important to seek out a medical doctor who is well trained and experienced in doing facial rejuvenation procedures.

Two

Choosing the Right Physician

Choosing the Right Physician

You've decided you want to do all you can to look and feel your best. And now you know that facial rejuvenation is possible without invasive surgery. But who should do it?

That's a crucial question. Because so many cosmetic procedures today are heavily hyped and marketed, it can be challenging to determine who is qualified—legally, ethically, and practically—to perform them. Next to a realistic appraisal of your needs, your wishes, and any risks involved, the single most important factor in your success is choosing a qualified professional.

Which Doctors Do Facial Rejuvenation?

Today the physicians who perform most skin rejuvenation procedures are facial plastic surgeons, plastic surgeons and dermatologists. It may be easy to find listings of physicians, but in the field of aesthetic surgery, it can be difficult for the consumer to sort out "who's who" from a bewildering mass of credentials. Many people are surprised to find out that any licensed medical doctor, regardless of training, can legally perform plastic surgery or claim the title "plastic surgeon." It is important that the physician you choose is certified by an appropriate board.

But what does being board-certified mean? According to the American Board of Medical Specialties, "a board-certified physician has completed an approved education training program and an evaluation process including an examination designed to assess the knowledge, skills, and experience necessary to provide quality patient care in that specialty."

After training and certification, a doctor's level of experience in the procedure you're considering is his or her single most important asset. Many of the procedures available today do not carry high risk for injury; however, other procedures do. For example, lasers are very powerful tools—some lasers vaporize human tissue at temperatures twice that of boiling water. These are great tools for resurfacing damaged skin, and the results can be remarkable. But such tools should be used only by physicians who have a great deal of experience with them.

Choose a physician who specializes in a procedure. Many plastic surgeons become expert in just two or three specific types of noninvasive treatment, which is a real advantage. For example, you probably wouldn't want a doctor to use a high-powered laser to resurface your facial skin if the doctor spends the biggest portion of his or her time doing *liposuction* of the abdomen. Sometimes, a doctor who claims enormous experience in every conceivable cutting-edge cosmetic technique may not be as wise a choice as one who has sought out extensive training in only a few procedures.

Plastic Surgeons

General plastic surgeons perform surgery involving the repair, reconstruction, or replacement of physical defects anywhere on the body. Some plastic surgeons specialize exclusively in cosmetic facial procedures. They offer surgical procedures such as facelifts as well as nonsurgical procedures.

In addition to medical school, general plastic surgeons spend three to five years of residency in general surgery, followed by two to three years of plastic surgery residency, which includes facial and cosmetic surgery as well as the repair of wounds or defects of the body, hands, and genitourinary tract. They are certified by the American Board of Plastic Surgery.

> *Plastic surgery is more than a doctor's technique. The doctor should be artistic, caring, and committed.*
>
> Michael Byun, M.D.
> Plastic Surgeon

Facial Plastic Surgeons

As the name suggests, facial plastic surgeons specialize in procedures for the face. They are qualified to perform both surgical and nonsurgical procedures of the face and neck.

13

Many also offer nonsurgical skin rejuvenation procedures.

Most facial plastic surgeons are *otolaryngologists*, or head and neck surgeons. After graduating from medical school, they spend one to two years in a general surgery residency, then four to five years in head and neck surgery, including facial plastic surgery, followed by a fellowship year in facial plastic and reconstructive surgery. They are certified by both the American Board of Otolaryngology Head and Neck Surgery and the American Board of Facial Plastic and Reconstructive Surgery upon successful completion of a certification examination.

Dermatologists and Dermatological Surgeons

Dermatologists and dermatological surgeons are physicians who treat disorders of the skin, hair, and nails, including skin cancers, hair loss, and scars, and skin changes associated with aging. Many also offer a variety of non-invasive cosmetic procedures such as chemical peels, dermabrasion, laser resurfacing, and the treatment of varicose veins.

Dermatologists must have graduated from an accredited medical school and completed a broad-based clinical residency program. In addition, they must have completed a three-year accredited dermatology residency program with at least 75 percent of their work being directly related to dermatology. After completing educational training, they are eligible for the certifying examination administered by the American Board of Dermatology or the American Board of Dermatological Surgery.

Other Staff and Assistants

Many physicians who perform cosmetic procedures employ highly trained physician assistants and registered nurses who perform procedures under the physician's supervision. Also, technicians, referred to as *estheticians*, perform "lighter" treatments such as facial steaming, mask applications, waxing, exfoliation, pore cleansing, and mild chemical peels.

Estheticians are licensed by the state; however, requirements vary widely from state to state. Some estheticians are trained by a variety of technical or cosmetology schools, others by physicians. Estheticians are not qualified to diagnose, or to perform any treatment that involves injections or that produces bleeding or oozing from the skin.

How to Find a Doctor

There are several ways you can maximize your chances of choosing a well-qualified professional who can help you achieve the results you're looking for. First, be proactive—educate yourself. Learn everything you can about the types of treatments available and which doctors in your community offer them. A good referral is a great place to begin. Here are some avenues for gathering information:

Word of mouth. Gather names from people you know who have had positive experiences with a certain doctor. Be sure they provide details on the results of their procedure, not just on the doctor's great personality or lovely office suite. Ask if they'd mind sharing their own before-and-after photos with you, and ask them to tell you what their procedure was like.

Your family doctor. Ask your primary physician to provide you with the names of plastic surgeons, facial plastic surgeons, or dermatologists he or she knows professionally or by reputation. Other health care professionals, including nurses, may also provide knowledgeable referrals.

Medical societies. These organizations can tell you who is, and is not, a member in good standing of local and regional medical societies and boards.

Local hospitals. Call hospitals in your area and ask for the names of doctors who have admitting privileges and who perform cosmetic procedures. If there is a nearby teaching hospital, ask which doctors are also involved in training other doctors in cosmetic procedures.

Spas. Today, many spas offer facial rejuvenation treatments; but is it safe to have a procedure done in a spa? Regulations for spas vary according to the state you live in, but the key point is whether the staff is experienced and well trained. Generally, it's a better idea to visit a doctor's office or clinic rather than a spa. The exception? When a spa has an on-staff

> *When you are in the office, you must be the most important person to the doctor and his/her staff. This will mark the difference between a competent result and an excellent result.*
>
> William Truswell, M.D.
> Facial Plastic Surgeon

M.D., such as a facial plastic surgeon, a plastic surgeon, a dermatologist, or another qualified physician. The spa's doctor should supervise any trained nurses or estheticians who perform the simplest procedures.

Your Consultation

After you've done your homework to find good referrals, don't hesitate to make consultation appointments with several different doctors. What's most important is to select a reputable specialist who will give you the best possible care. Even though these rejuvenation procedures are not surgical, they are medical. Your doctor should be thorough in assessing whether or not you should have a procedure. The purpose of the first consultation with a doctor is to:

- establish trust and communication

- allow the doctor to take a medical history

- establish your needs

- explain options to you

- inform you about treatment outcomes

It's important that you feel at ease with your doctor, and especially that you sense you are being advised realistically and appropriately about what to expect from a procedure. Although most non-invasive cosmetic treatments involve minimal risks, risks do exist, and a doctor who takes a thorough medical history and carefully explains any risks has your best interests in mind. Honesty and confidence are good; arrogance and wild promises are not. Trust your instincts—if you feel you're receiving thorough information with sensitivity to your needs and concerns, you're probably in the right place.

Questions to Ask During Your Consultation

Which cosmetic procedures do you perform on a regular basis, and how many?

If a doctor claims to do a procedure "all the time," ask for more details. For example, a doctor who has done only a dozen of the procedure you're considering is still on the learning curve. But if the answer is at least a dozen a month, that's a better indicator of solid experience. The largest practices might do over 100 microdermabrasions or chemical peels a month, for example.

Where would my procedure be performed—in your office or in a hospital?

Most non-invasive procedures are performed in the doctor's office. You'll sit in a chair similar to a dentist's chair, with a comfortable headrest. Unless the skin of your upper chest is also being treated, there's no need to disrobe. A gown will be given to you to wear over your clothing. The few procedures that work on your skin at a deeper level, such as complete laser resurfacing or a deep chemical peel, or others that require *intravenous (IV) sedation* or *twilight anesthesia*, are done on a surgical table in a hospital or surgical suite, with sterile draping and other infection control precautions, just as would be done for any surgery.

Has your office or clinic been certified by the American Accreditation Association for Ambulatory Healthcare or the American Association for Ambulatory Plastic Surgery Facilities?

Because many surgeons who perform cosmetic procedures work in large practices that incorporate freestanding surgical suites, it's important to know that these facilities meet quality standards. Certification by either of these organizations ensures that the surgical area is regularly reviewed and inspected for standards including the facility's general and operating room environments; policy and procedures; general safety in the facility; blood and medications handling; medical records; quality assessment and improvement; and personnel. These organizations also provide standardized practice guidelines for the surgeon operating in single-specialty ambulatory surgical facilities.

Would any of your patients who have had the procedure I am considering be willing to talk to me?

The doctor should be willing to put you in touch with another patient who is willing to be interviewed. To respect their confidentiality, the doctor will not give you another patient's name and phone number, but more likely will ask a patient who's willing to talk to contact you. You might ask the former patient:

- Were the doctor and his or her staff compassionate and supportive?

- Did you feel you had been given ample information before the procedure?

- Did you have any pain, and if so, how was it managed?

- Were there any problems with your procedure, and if so, how were they corrected?

- Were you satisfied with the outcome?

- Would you continue if this procedure requires repeated treatments?

May I see actual before-and-after photos, not brochures, showing patients you have treated?

As in any other publication, photos in brochures can be airbrushed, and special lighting and makeup can exaggerate the transformations between "before" and "after." An actual photograph is likely to give you a better idea of what you can expect. Keep in mind that individual results will vary, depending on each person's skin condition, age, and level of skin damage, as well as on the type of treatment.

What are the potential risks with this procedure?

Even though risks may seem minimal, ask about them. How often do they occur? And if they do occur, how are they handled? Avoid any physician who is not willing to thoroughly explain risks and how they are handled.

What will the recovery period be like?

Sometimes we may get caught up in the excitement about the results of a procedure and may forget about recovery time. Nonsurgical procedures do not typically require the same type of recovery we associate with invasive surgery; however, some procedures will mean some down time for you. Ask about any restrictions and how soon you can return to work or other activities.

What is the physician's policy on "surgical" revisions?

This question mostly refers to surgical procedures. Sometimes after a surgical procedure is performed, an additional procedure, a "revision," is needed to achieve the final result. However, it is possible for a nonsurgical procedure require follow-up attention. Ask how the doctor handles such matters. Is there additional cost for any follow-up treatment?

What is the cost of the procedure?

It is important to clearly establish the cost for your procedure. Insurance does not pay for elective, cosmetic procedures, and most physicians require payment in advance. The cost to you covers such things as fees for the surgeon, surgical suite, and anesthesiologist, if one is required. Other costs might include those for blood tests and medications.

Costs vary for nonsurgical facial rejuvenation procedures, based on geographical location. For example, a chemical peel in New York City will likely cost more than one in the Midwest.

American Attitudes about Cosmetic Surgery

- More than half of Americans, 54 percent, approve of cosmetic surgery. Twenty-four percent say they could consider having a cosmetic procedure.

- Nearly one-third of women, 30 percent, say they would consider cosmetic surgery, compared to 18 percent of men.

- Nearly 75 percent of men and women say they would not be embarrassed if others knew that they were having a cosmetic procedure.

Survey by the American Society for Aesthetic Plastic Surgery, 2003

Three

Botox Injections

Botox Injections

In the past few years, Botox injections have topped the list as the most popular nonsurgical facial rejuvenation procedure. It seems an unlikely use for a chemical first discovered by ophthalmologists almost twenty years ago to treat two eye muscle disorders: uncontrollable blinking (*blepharospasm*) and misaligned eyes (*strabismus*). The ophthalmologists began to notice an unexpected side effect: the frown lines between their patients' eyebrows seemed to vanish, their foreheads smoothed, and even their crow's feet were less evident. In April 2002, the Food and Drug Administration (FDA) officially approved Botox for treating frown lines between the eyes. What makes Botox so popular is that the injections are quick and easy to repeat.

Botox is actually a protein produced by the *botulinum* bacterium, that causes a form of food poisoning. That may sound alarming, but you cannot contract botulism from the tiny amount of toxin present in a Botox injection, because it is sterilized and highly purified.

What Botox Does

Botox eliminates dynamic wrinkles, those that form as a result of facial expressions, by paralyzing the underlying muscles which contract and cause the wrinkle. What is the science behind this? Normally, your brain sends electrical messages to your muscles to tell them to contract. These messages are transmitted by a chemical neurotransmitter called *acetylcholine.* When Botox is injected into the muscles just beneath the skin, it blocks this chemical's release. As a result, the message to contract never reaches the muscles. Since the muscles aren't moving, the creases they

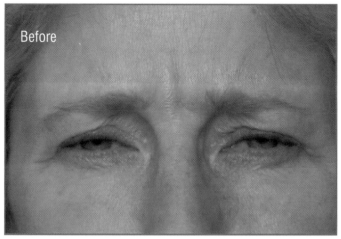

Patient making frown expression before Botox injections.

normally create are no longer visible. A smoother skin surface and more relaxed look are the results.

Wrinkles Treated with Botox

Frown Lines

Botox is best known for erasing frown lines—the creases that appear between the eyebrows, medically known as the *glabella* region. Not only will the injections stop the repeated muscle contractions that make you look constantly annoyed or tired (even when you're not), but they can also prevent the surface, static wrinkles there from deepening.

Furrowed Foreheads

Perhaps you've developed a worried or even melancholy appearance. This may be due to deep, horizontal forehead wrinkles that appear when you're puzzled or concerned, or simply because you've had a long-standing habit of raising your eyebrows. Botox injections beneath these furrows will prevent these lines from forming, leaving you with a more serene, relaxed-looking brow.

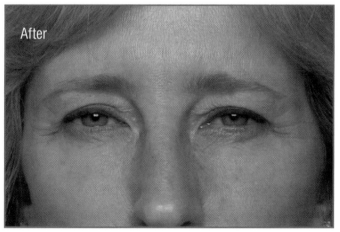

Patient making frown expression after Botox injections. Muscles in the glabella region, between the eyes, do not respond.

23

Crow's Feet

Botox injections can greatly reduce the appearance of crow's feet—the fine lines that appear at the corners of your eyes when you smile or squint. If treatments are continued, the relaxed muscles may never return to their original state, which means you may have a sustained smoothed effect.

Other Wrinkles

Botox can diminish "lipstick" or "smoker's" lines in the upper lip caused by repeated mouth pursing. Likewise, lines that run straight down from the corners of the mouth can be softened. Such lines are known as "marionette" lines—think of the famous puppet Howdy

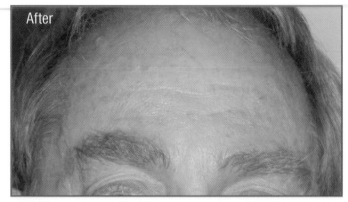

Eyebrows raised after Botox injections. Forehead muscles stay relaxed.

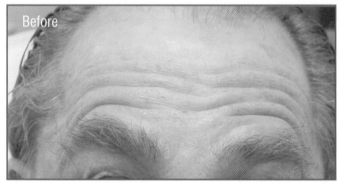

Eyebrows raised, creating lines in forehead, before Botox injections.

Doody's chin. Sometimes, Botox is also used to treat vertical neck wrinkles caused by subtle muscle movements, though these are not considered "expression" lines.

Combined with Other Treatments

In areas where Botox can't completely eliminate a wrinkle, it is often used in combination with other line-smoothing treatments, such as chemical peels, filler injections, laser treatments, or microdermabrasion. Your doctor can create a wrinkle-fighting strategy that includes Botox as part of a broader treatment plan. For example, for upper lip lines, a chemical peel or laser resurfacing might be the primary approach, with Botox added to prevent the lines from re-forming.

Are You a Candidate for Botox?

Botox is a safe procedure for the vast majority of people. Some people, however, have conditions that make it an unwise choice.

Your doctor needs to determine whether you have allergies to any of the components in the Botox solution, including albumin (a blood-derived protein), glucose, or yeast; the injections might trigger an allergic response, although this is very unusual. A more common issue is that Botox can interact with some medications, so it's important to be sure your doctor knows about any drugs you are taking. In particular, calcium channel blockers, quinine, penicillamine, and the antibiotics known as aminoglycosides do not mix safely with Botox. Botox can unpredictably intensify these medications' effects, meaning that the dosage your doctor has prescribed might suddenly have a more powerful effect.

Botox injections are not recommended for women while they are pregnant or breast-feeding. Some muscle-weakening conditions will also rule out Botox. For example, if you have multiple sclerosis, myasthenia gravis, Lou Gehrig's disease, or Bell's palsy, you are not a candidate for Botox treatment. Your doctor will review your health history thoroughly before agreeing that Botox is right for you.

Preparing for Botox Injections

Since Botox is simply an injection, there is no advance preparation needed. One exception can be that your doctor may advise you to stop taking certain supplements, such as garlic, gingko biloba, or ginseng, for two weeks beforehand, since these can increase the possibility of bruising at the injection sites. Likewise, if you are taking blood-thinners, which may also increase the possibility of bruising, your doctor will want to discuss these medications with your prescribing physician. You should never stop taking an important medicine for a cosmetic procedure, however (and after all, most bruising can be covered with makeup).

You may want to bring in photos of yourself at a younger age and photos of an older relative you may resemble to your first consultation. These can help you and your doctor determine which areas you want to have treated. If your discussion indicates that you are a good candidate and there are no pressing reasons to wait, it is often possible to receive your Botox treatments on your first visit. You'll want to schedule your "Botox day" at least two full days before an important event.

How Is Botox Injected?

Most of our Botox patients are women, but more men are getting injections. We do a ton of Botox injections, and about 80% of our patients return for repeat treatments once they've seen the result.

Kirsten
Surgical technician

A Botox injection is a simple procedure. What won't be as simple is the selection of injection sites. The doctor will base decisions not only on how your face looks on the outside, but also on the underlying muscles that create your wrinkles from within. Based on these observations, the doctor knows where to insert the needles and how much Botox solution to use for each injection.

Before the injections, your skin is cleaned with alcohol. Then, a bright light will be directed on your face to allow your doctor to highlight creases and shadows. Most patients don't require anesthesia; however, you may be offered an ice pack for about five minutes, to numb your skin, or a topical numbing cream, which takes about thirty minutes to take effect. Some people skip the cream because the short, thin needles used with Botox mean these injections are less painful than most other shots and cause only a slight burning sensation. Other patients simply don't want to take the extra time required for the anesthetic. It's an individual decision.

Your doctor may ask you to grin, scowl, grimace, or make other expressions. While you're forming these expressions, your doctor will press on areas of your face to determine the location of the dynamic wrinkles; he or she needs to feel the muscle thickness in order to determine the best points to inject.

For the areas most commonly treated, the number of injections required per treatment will vary. It all depends on your own pattern and depth of wrinkling. In the glabella or "frown line" region, usually five to seven injections will do. For crow's feet, two to seven are given on each side. And in the forehead, from eight to fifteen or more injections may be needed. In some places, your doctor may gently massage the area to distribute the solution.

The average Botox injection procedure takes about five to seven minutes, depending on how many areas you're having treated. Afterward, you may be offered an ice compress for about a minute to minimize redness at the injection sites. Then, you're ready to go.

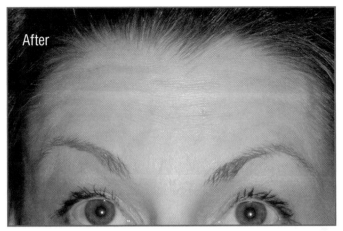

Eyebrows lifted after Botox injections.

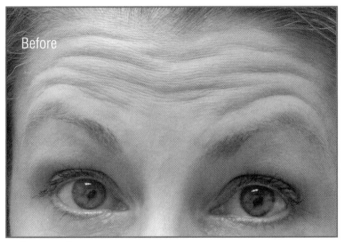

Lifting eyebrows prior to Botox injections.

How Will I Look?

Immediately after your Botox injections, you'll have little red bumps at each injection site. This slight swelling is about the size of a mosquito bite. The vast majority of the time these will subside—within just an hour or two, which is why many people schedule their treatments during a lunch hour. Occasionally, however, very subtle swelling might linger for a day or two.

It will take anywhere from several days to a few weeks for you to see and feel the full results of your Botox treatments. That's because the nerves within your muscles already contain some amount of acetylcholine (the chemical that Botox blocks) and it takes time for the existing supply to dissipate. Once that happens, the Botox effect begins.

Some people notice a dramatic change with Botox. Others find that they're hearing lots of comments on how terrific they look. Again, it all depends on your "situation." You'll certainly see the difference yourself. You'll have smoother skin, fewer or shallower wrinkles, and a more relaxed and rested look. Because Botox is so subtle, it can bring youthful changes to your face without anyone guessing why. Sometimes, people might just observe that you seem to be "in a really good mood."

> *I had a Botox injection for the vertical frown line between my eyebrows. It totally relaxed that "crease." After my husband saw the result, he went in for an injection, too.*
>
> Ginny, 54

Follow-Up Care

After Botox injections, follow-up is uncomplicated. There are a few basic cautions your doctor will go over with you. First, do not rub the places that were injected for twenty-four hours, as you don't want the Botox to spread into areas not intended for treatment.

Also, some doctors advise that you avoid lying flat and stay upright or in a seated position for three or four hours; others think that's overkill. Those who do suggest staying upright want to ensure that any yet-unabsorbed Botox can't drift into other muscles of your face. This is a very unlikely prospect, however. Most doctors agree that after your appointment you can behave as you normally would and that the risk of "Botox budge" is minimal.

If you do have any bruising at the injection sites, a bag of frozen peas or a small ice pack, wrapped in a towel and applied for about twenty minutes, will help relieve it. You can repeat the ice pack application once an hour for several hours, as needed.

How Long Will Results Last?

The effects of Botox are temporary, lasting approximately three to four months for most people. Many who are delighted with the procedure decide to have repeated treatments to maintain the effect. And, patients who receive another treatment before the previous treatment stops working find that the results last six to eight months.

If there's anything you don't like about your Botox results, however, they are entirely reversible. As the toxin's effect ebbs from the muscles, you'll notice a gradual return of the dynamic wrinkles. Because the change is subtle and slow, you can schedule renewal treatments at approximately four-month intervals. However, some people find that injections twice a year maintain their smooth new look.

A bonus to Botox treatment is its gradual effect on the static lines over the deeper, dynamic ones. As muscles stay loose and relaxed in an area where they used to contract, deepening of the static lines is halted. Your body also has time to gradually bring collagen and other surface-building substances to the area of the finer lines, where over time the skin has thinned. So if Botox injections are continued at regular intervals, even though Botox itself is temporary, over time the treatment contributes to permanent wrinkle smoothing.

Potential Risks

Botox has an outstanding safety record. As with any procedure, however, there are some statistical risks. A small percentage of people who've had forehead wrinkles treated will develop a headache, for an evening or possibly several days. On occasion, again with the treatment of the forehead, if too much toxin is injected or the area is rubbed too hard, a "droopy" brow can result. And if improper technique is used near the eyes, there's a very small risk (2 to 5 percent) that a temporary droopy eyelid might result. This problem would disappear in a few weeks, however. Great care is required when using Botox near the mouth, because if mouth muscles are overweakened that can conceivably cause drooling or difficulty in speaking clearly. These potential risks are reversible, however, and would diminish as the Botox wears off.

> *I had Botox for the frown line between my eyes. It worked so well, I had injections in my "crow's feet." It was quick and painless. I will go back for more treatments when it's time.*
>
> Lori, 48

Botox Parties

One method of marketing Botox has sprung up that should be considered with great care: Botox parties, bashes or other group treatment events. For some time, promoters have been offering parties that provide discount rates and a party atmosphere, even including wine. It has become the "hot" new way to try Botox.

Those events can backfire, however. Do you really want to make a decision about a cosmetic treatment under the influence of pressure from excited friends, or possibly after you have had an alcoholic drink, which may impair your judgment? To be safe, attend group events only if they are information seminars. Then schedule an appointment with the doctor for a consultation and treatment.

Although getting a Botox injection may sound as simple as getting a flu shot from a friendly nurse, it's not. Only licensed physicians with special training in the procedure should be allowed anywhere near your face with a Botox needle. That's because to get the proper effect from Botox, your doctor must take a thorough health history and make a careful

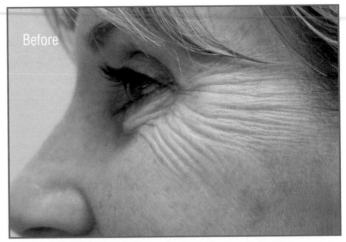

"Crow's feet" around eyes before Botox injections.

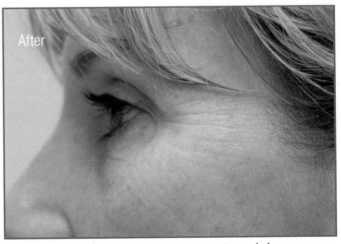

Three weeks after Botox injections around the corners of the eyes.

assessment of your individual wrinkling patterns and facial musculature. Facial anatomy is complex, and this assessment is something that not even a registered nurse is sufficiently trained to do. The injection technique requires delicacy, precision, and a great deal of specialized medical knowledge.

Questions to Ask Your Doctor

- Is Botox appropriate for me?

- Are most of my wrinkles dynamic or static?

- What kind of results do you expect from Botox in my case?

- Should I be considering other wrinkle treatments, too?

- Will I need pain medication?

- How soon will I see my results?

- Can you show me before-and-after photos of other patients?

- How should I care for my skin before and after the injections?

- Should I stop taking my usual medications or supplements?

Four

Chemical Peels

Chemical Peels

Would you like to "peel away" a few years and have smoother, softer, fresher-looking skin? If so, a *chemical peel* may be right for you. Chemical peels are the oldest method of facial rejuvenation. It's reported that chemical peels were popular in ancient Egypt; the Egyptians used sand in lotions they concocted to exfoliate the skin.

Certainly, the process has evolved since ancient times. For the last fifty years, doctors have used new and improved peeling agents to renew aging skin. Most of these procedures are quick, healing is relatively rapid, and the results can make a remarkable difference.

What Peels Do

The solution in a chemical peel removes the top layer of skin, leaving your face smoother and fresher. Peels restore sun-damaged skin. They also diminish wrinkles, acne scars, and can improve irregularities in the skin tone. For example, a peel can eliminate discoloration such as *melasma*, the brown patches that often accompany pregnancy. Peels will also eliminate age spots and the yellowish bumps called *solar elastosis*, which are areas of degenerated collagen caused by sun exposure. Peels can remove the precancerous lesions known as *actinic keratoses*.

Although a chemical peel can soften the appearance of deep wrinkles, such as nasolabial folds and frown lines, it will not totally remove them. A peel won't tighten skin, but because it improves its surface and texture, your skin may appear firmer. Some research indicates that peels boost collagen production, which may help forestall the formation of new wrinkles.

Modern formulas for chemical peels contain a blend of ingredients that offer additional benefits. For example, a peel formula may contain hormones, anti-acne agents, or melanin inhibitors. Hormones enhance the plumpness of the skin by increasing moisture content. Anti-acne ingredients kill bacteria and absorb excess oils. Melanin inhibitors help prohibit the formation of skin discoloration or brown spots.

Types of Peels

Light Peels

The most popular peel is the *light peel* or *superficial peel*. These peels remove the top layer of skin—the dead surface cells, called the *stratum corneum*. The chemical solutions in these peels are *alpha hydroxy acids (AHAs)*. Most of these acids are derived from citrus fruits, milk sugars, and sugar cane. The mildest of the peel formulas, AHAs brighten, freshen, and exfoliate skin, repairing minor sun damage and smoothing dry areas. Because AHAs remove only the most superficial layer of the skin, healing is so swift that these are sometimes called "weekend" peels. Many people will have a light peel done on a Friday,

---

Chemical Peels Improve:

- Fine lines and wrinkles
- Uneven pigmentation
- Shallow acne scars
- Sun-damaged skin
- Age spots
- Freckling

---

and return to work on Monday, with minimal makeup.

Medium Peels

For a medium peel, a more potent chemical is used to remove all of the outer skin layer, or epidermis. The chemical, *trichloroacetic acid (TCA)*, is a colorless synthetic acid, normally used in a concentration of about 35 percent. Because it penetrates more deeply than a light peel, a medium peel goes further to rejuvenate sun-damaged skin. Medium peels also reduce fine surface lines and wrinkles, often completely removing them. A medium peel is particularly effective at treating uneven

35

pigment, such as age spots or melasma. It will also diminish superficial blemishes and shallow scarring from acne, but not deep, "pitted" scars.

Depending on your skin's condition and what you'd like to have treated, your doctor may combine your medium peel with a simultaneous light peel. After the AHA exfoliates the most superficial layer of your skin, the TCA penetrates more deeply, maximizing the benefits.

> *Patients usually have the most wrinkles around the eyes and mouth. So, I may adjust the chemical solution and do a slightly deeper peel in these areas and a lighter peel on the rest of the face.*
>
> Dr. Jon Mendelsohn
> Facial Plastic Surgeon

Deep Peels

The traditional deep peel procedure which you may have heard about over the years uses a chemical called *phenol*, sometimes referred to as carbolic acid. A deep peel removes all of the epidermis and part of the skin's middle layer, the dermis. As a result, it removes wrinkles around the mouth and eyes. Creases in the nasolabial fold and deep crow's feet soften but do not disappear totally.

Since the risks, recovery, and complications are higher with a traditional phenol peel,

a newer procedure, a *modified deep peel* is rapidly growing in popularity. For this procedure, the peel solution ingredients—liquid soap, Croton oil, phenol, and water—are modified. The modification uses less Croton oil, which enhances the effect, but eliminates the complications and potential toxicity frequently associated with the deeper peels.

You may hear this newer peel referred to as a Hetter Peel, named for Dr. Gregory Hetter, its inventor. It is also called a Croton oil peel, or a modified phenol peel. The effects of modified deep peel are dramatic when used for facial wrinkling, especially the leathery criss-cross lines, and deep lines around the lips, so common with sun damage.

The deeper peels can be done in localized areas such as under the eyes, for "crepey" lower lids, or around the mouth to remove the vertical "smoker's lines." Or it can be used on the entire face for an overall skin rejuvenation.

Are You a Candidate for a Peel?

If you simply want to smooth and refresh tired-looking skin, you're likely a candidate for

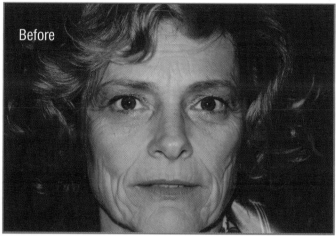

Wrinkles before full-face deep peel.

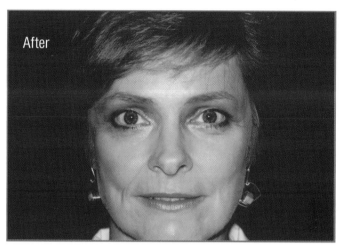

Three to four months after deep peel.

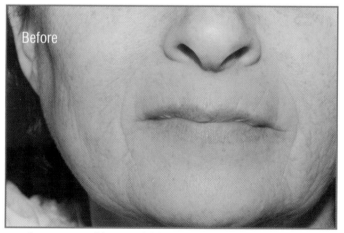

Moderate wrinkles and blotchy skin patches.

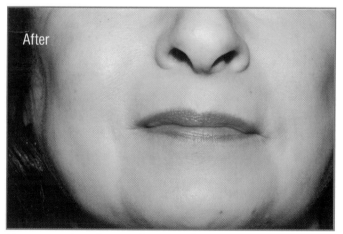

Four months after medium peel.

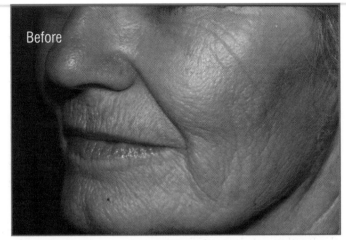

Facial wrinkles and vertical lines above upper lip.

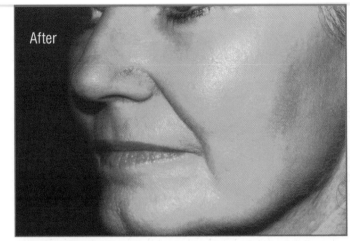

Four months after deep peel.

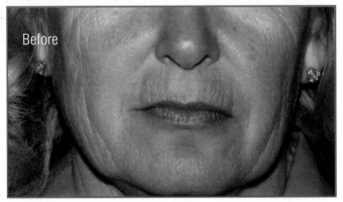

Wrinkles and sun-damaged skin.

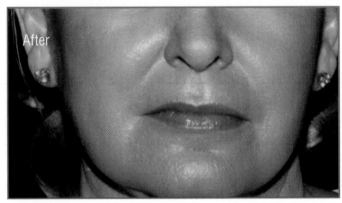

Several months after deep peel.

a light peel performed by a qualified physician. Likewise, if you have dark or black skin, your best choice is a light peel, because it is less likely to cause any pigmentation change. Most people can work these peels into their schedules with minimal time off from work.

If you're fair-skinned you may also be a good candidate for a medium peel. For medium-toned or dark skin there is some risk of irregular pigmentation, however. Be aware that healing can take up to two weeks, so you may want to plan a short vacation around your scheduled procedure.

Modified deep peels are recommended only for people with fair skin—they are not advisable for medium, dark, black, or very oily skin. Recovery may take one to two weeks, with redness lasting up to six months.

Preparing for Your Peel

If you are using *Retin-A* (*retinoic acid*), or a similar product, as part of a skin care regimen, you should stop using it for two to three days prior to your peel. The technician doing the peel should be made aware of your Retin-A use since it will affect the penetration of the peel solution. Otherwise, cleansing is the only preparation needed for a light peel. You simply wash your face with the cleanser provided at your doctor's office when you arrive.

In contrast, for a medium peel or deeper peel, your doctor may recommend that you pretreat your skin for several weeks with a prescription cream such as Retin-A. This exfoliates the skin and allows the solution to penetrate more deeply. Your doctor will instruct you on whether you need to discontinue using the Retin-A before your peel. If one of your problems is dark spots or blotchiness, a bleaching cream, *hydroquinone*, might also be added to boost your skin's pretreatment conditioning. This cream suppresses the melanin in the skin, causing dark spots to lighten; using the cream also lessens the risk of pigmentation problems after the peel. If you tend to get cold sores, your doctor will prescribe prophylactic (preventative) antiviral medications to suppress

> *Chemical peels are effective for removing wrinkles and sun damage in the skin under the eyes. A peel can accomplish more in these areas than plastic surgery.*
>
> Jon Mendelsohn
> Facial Plastic Surgeon

any new outbreak, which might spread from the lips into a treated facial area.

Before a deep peel, you'll need a medical checkup. Any patient who plans to undergo anesthesia should be checked for heart, kidney, liver, or lung problems; the procedure carries a slightly increased risk for those with such problems.

Stop smoking for at least a week before your appointment, and avoid alcohol. Both will impede healing—smoking constricts blood vessels and alcohol dehydrates your tissues, which need their natural fluids for repair. Start taking your antibiotics as instructed. These are prescribed because a modified deep peel leaves dermal tissue exposed, and as with any wound to the skin, it's important to prevent infection. Arrange for someone to drive you home afterward and help you for forty-eight hours; you may be lightheaded from the residual anesthesia.

Before a medium or deep peel, your doctor may have you stop certain medications for several weeks. *Anticoagulant,* or blood thinning, medicines or herbal supplements may make it harder to recover, because your blood

brings healing nutrients to the raw skin. Most doctors also recommend that if you're taking drugs known as *oral retinoids,* used to treat skin conditions such as severe acne or psoriasis, you stop these for six months before a deep peel. These drugs, which include Accutane, can slow new skin formation, and they can also increase the risk of scarring.

How Is a Peel Performed?

All peels involve solutions applied to the skin, but details vary according to the type of peel. Every peel is applied with attention to your individual skin tone, condition, and level of damage. Your doctor will carefully control the depth of penetration for the best results.

Usually, peels are done on the entire face. With the deeper peels, the depth of the peel is usually greater around the eyes and mouth since more wrinkles are usually present in these areas. Sometimes partial peels, or "sub units" of the face, are done when only a portion of the facial skin is damaged and in need of repair. However, such a partial peel may leave a line of demarcation between the treated and nontreated regions.

Light Peel

A light peel is performed in your doctor's office. After you've washed your face, your doctor or a technician uses a solvent such as alcohol or diluted acetone to remove every remaining trace of makeup or oil. In some practices, the doctor may pretreat your skin with a simple, painless procedure called *dermaplaning,* which lightly abrades the skin surface to remove dead skin cells and aid in the penetration of the chemicals. This is usually done by passing a bladed instrument that resembles an electric razor over your skin. Some doctors use a blade, similar to a scalpel.

Then the AHA solution is evenly applied, usually with a cotton pad or brush. You'll feel stinging, but it is usually not uncomfortable enough to require pain medication. The solution is left on your skin for about seven minutes. If your doctor uses glycolic acid, a chemical that penetrates more readily than other AHAs, it is then rinsed thoroughly with saline solution to neutralize its action and prevent harm to the skin. The other AHAs do not require rinsing. Finally, moisturizing cream is applied to your face.

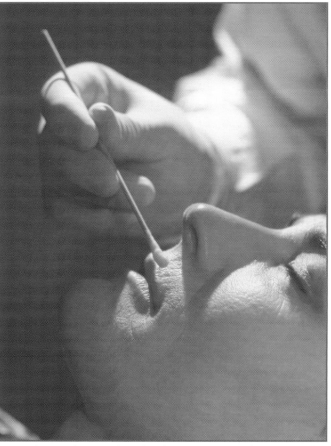

A medium chemical peel solution is applied. Notice the skin turning a frosty white on the side of the patient's face.

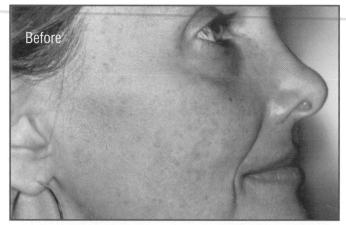

Prior to a medium peel to even the skin tone.

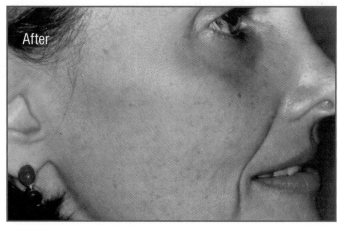

Several weeks after medium peel.

Medium Peel

Like a light peel, a medium peel is performed in your physician's office. Your skin is cleansed and your doctor applies the solution to your face with a surgical sponge, which usually takes about ten to fifteen minutes. In about forty-five seconds, the chemical solution will cause your skin to temporarily turn a white, frosty color. This reaction is caused by the solution removing the surface skin cells.

Finally, you may sit under a fan for a while to help cool the burn. The burning sensation is stronger with a medium peel, so your doctor may suggest taking a mild sedative and ibuprofen beforehand.

Deep Peel

A deep peel or modified deep peel is usually done with twilight or general anesthesia in an accredited surgical facility. The patient's heart is monitored throughout the procedure; if too much phenol penetrates too deeply and enters the blood stream, it could cause heart rhythm disturbances.

Once you are asleep, or comfortably dozy, your skin is cleansed, and a solvent is used to

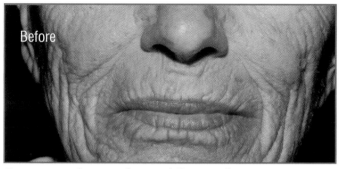

Severe sun damage from a lifetime of exposure to sun.

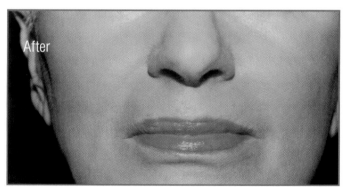

Three to four months after deep peel.

remove surface oil, enabling the solution to penetrate evenly. The peel solution is applied with applicator sticks, focusing on the areas with the most damage. A lighter application is applied to the other areas, taking care to blend the areas and "feather" the edges to prevent lines of demarcation. The entire procedure takes from fifteen minutes to one hour, depending on how much of the face is treated.

Once the procedure is over, your doctor will cover your face with an emollient cream or petroleum jelly. The cream seals the skin, retaining moisture and preventing scab formation and scarring. When you awaken, the sensation is similar to a serious sunburn, easily relieved with pain medication After you rest for an hour or two in the recovery area, you'll be ready to go home with your driver.

How Will I Look?

Light Peel

For the next few days after a light peel your skin is likely to be somewhat pink, and you may notice some mild dryness or flakiness. All these effects are easily camouflaged with light makeup, however, and soon you'll be aware only that your skin is fresher and smoother, and that you're looking more rested than usual.

Medium Peel

After a medium peel, your skin will turn red, darken, peel, and in some cases, may (or may not) develop some soft scabbed areas—better described as soft crusts—during the next several days. Crusting will depend on your skin condition and response to the treatment. The areas that received the greatest penetration of acid will be more likely to crust over.

> *I had crow's feet and a lot of sun damage. My chemical peel took ten years off my face.*
> Tammy, 39

You'll probably not want to go out. It usually takes up to seven to ten days to feel presentable again, although with makeup, you may feel comfortable after a week. Your skin color will gradually fade from red to a light pink. Once your new skin emerges, most of your fine wrinkles and blotches will have disappeared.

You shouldn't experience much discomfort, but if you do, ask your doctor for pain medication. Take the medication as needed over the next few days.

Deep Peel

The good news is that a deeper peel produces remarkable results. The bad news? You'll look a whole lot worse before you look better. After the peel, your face will be very swollen for a day or so. During the first week, the swelling will be followed by peeling like that from a severe sunburn. Parts of your face will ooze.

Many patients report they don't have a lot of pain after this peel; however, they often report a burning sensation for the first six to eight hours. Keeping the entire face moist with prescribed creams will prevent pain. Your doctor will prescribe mild pain medication, which you may wish to use, depending on how you're feeling.

You may find it uncomfortable to make facial movements. So, you may not feel like talking for the first few days, and you may be more comfortable drinking liquids and eating soft foods, which require less chewing.

Usually after six to eight days, if you had any crusting, most of it will be gone. Your face will be very red, but you can begin to cover the redness with makeup. About a month after the procedure, your new skin will feel rough or even finely wrinkled. This will smooth out over the next six to eight weeks, and the redness will fade to baby-skin pink. The risk of permanent change in pigmentation is less with a modified deep peel, compared to the original deep peels. Your new skin is likely to be somewhat lighter, though a darker shade is also possible. If your entire face has been peeled, any overall color change is less likely to be noticeable.

Follow-Up Care

After any peel, the number one commitment you must make to your new complexion—permanently—is to protect it from the sun. We'll discuss how to do this in detail in chapter 9, but two sunscreen facts bear repeating: use copious amounts. For example, use a large marble-sized dollop for your face and three marbles-sized dollops for your neck and upper chest. Wait thirty minutes after applying it before you go out. Meanwhile, here's how to care for your face after a peel.

Light Peel

The flaking and dryness that follow an AHA peel are temporary and easily soothed with rich moisturizers and generous daily applications of a good, high-SPF sunscreen. Beyond that there's no new limit on your daily skin routine; you can wear no makeup or as much as you wish.

Medium Peel

Avoid scratching or picking at your face and any crusts that may develop. Cleanse gently using the products your doctor provides for you to take home. Washing with water may be too drying, and your doctor will want you to protect your skin with appropriate cleansers and ointments. Avoid the sun completely for as long as possible, and once you do go out, never skip your full-spectrum sunblock.

Deep Peel

During the first five to ten days after your peel, you will need to keep the peel area covered with emollient cream or petroleum jelly, prescribed by your doctor. The peeled area must remain moist at all times, until the oozing stops.

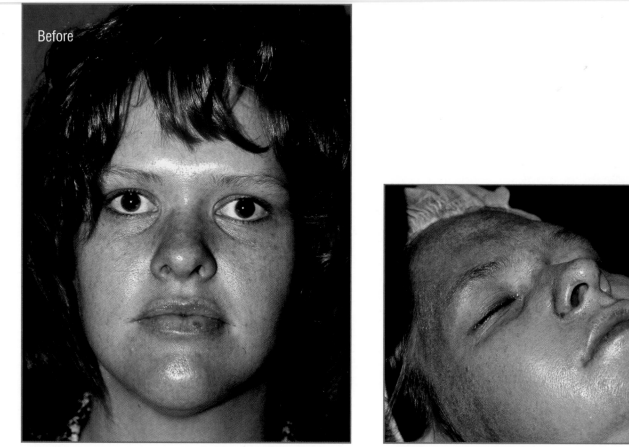

This 27-year-old woman wanted a chemical peel to diminish freckles and patches of blotchy skin.

A medium peel, an Obaji Blue Peel, has been applied. Note the even blue frost.

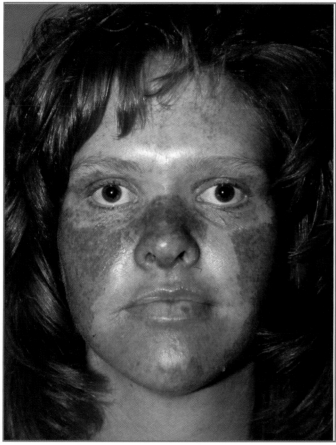

Three days after the peel, the skin begins to slough.

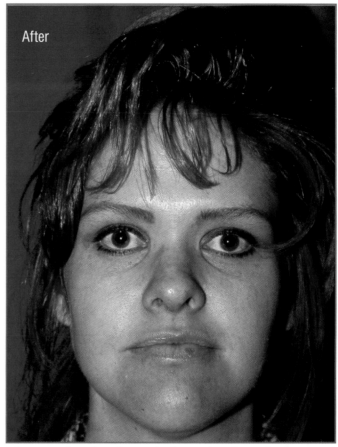

After

Three weeks after the peel. Skin is brighter, fresher, and skin tone is even.

Keeping the skin moist will prevent the skin from drying or crusting, which will create scarring. Also, avoid scarring by picking or scratching your face as it heals.

To cleanse your face, gently use your fingertips and cool water. Pat your face dry with a clean towel and apply the cream your doctor has ordered. You'll need to continue this washing and moisturizing for seven to ten days. Your doctor will tell you when it's safe to wear makeup again, and what cleansers and cosmetics to use.

For at least two months, postpone sports and recreation that expose you to the sun; ease slowly back into your exercise routine; and plan on wearing sunblock forever.

Sleep on extra pillows until the swelling subsides. Keeping your head elevated will encourage the dissipation of the excess fluids that have collected in the tissue of your face.

How Long Will Results Last?

Some people elect to repeat light peels every few weeks, but most doctors advise two- to three-month intervals. If light peels are done too often, they will dry the skin. Dryness promotes wrinkles. (The exception to having a light peel every few weeks may be using a very light glycolic acid solution that is applied weekly for about six weeks, for the cumulative effect of a light peel.)

Medium and deep peels last much longer. Although you might repeat a medium peel after one year if you have still not obtained the results you were aiming for, in most cases and with proper skin care, you're more likely to wait for years. Since modified deep peels remove the entire top layer of your facial skin, they produce permanent changes and a completely new skin surface.

Potential Risks

There are few risks with a light peel, other than possible lingering dryness. If you have had cold sores recently, a few weeks of antibiotic use beforehand is advisable. If the herpes simplex virus that triggers cold sores is currently active in your skin, the peel could trigger a new outbreak, with a risk of infection and scarring.

With medium peels, there is some risk of permanent scarring, pigmentation change, uneven texture, or demarcation lines. These are uncommon complications when you're in the hands of a highly experienced professional. Infection is also a potential risk. Closely following your doctor's aftercare instructions greatly reduces your risk of infection. Your doctor may also prescribe an antibiotic.

Deeper peels can cause heart rhythm disturbance and lasting kidney damage in some people if too much phenol enters the skin. Careful medical monitoring during the procedure should prevent problems. As with medium peels, permanent skin pigmentation changes, in which skin color becomes paler or uneven, are also possible.

Questions to Ask Your Doctor

- What type of peel is appropriate for me?

- How quickly will I recover?

- Can you show me before-and-after photos of other patients?

- How should I care for my skin before and after the peel?

- Should I stop taking my usual medications or supplements?

Five

Laser Skin Treatments

Laser Skin Treatments

Lasers are among the most powerful, advanced technologies on earth. Manufacturers use them to cut through steel. Doctors use them to cut through human tissue in delicate surgeries. In fact, today lasers have a wide range of applications in medicine and have become useful tools in facial rejuvenation. Lasers can "zap" away imperfections such as age spots and excess facial hair. Or they can be used to "resurface" the entire face, erasing fine lines and wrinkles.

How does a laser work on the skin? A laser produces a narrow beam, or wave of light, which emits an intense heat. Targeted at the skin, the laser can eliminate or reduce skin imperfections in a fraction of a second without damaging surrounding tissue. Because the laser beam is computer-driven, the depth of the beam's penetration into the skin is controlled.

Two basic types of lasers are used to treat skin: ablative and non-ablative. Ablative lasers, the more "aggressive" of the two, are capable of ablating, or completely removing, a layer of skin. The results are similar to that of a deep chemical peel, and in some cases, are almost as effective as a surgical facelift. Non-ablative lasers are less aggressive and are used for a variety of cosmetic purposes.

What Ablative Lasers Do

Ablative lasers are used to resurface the skin, the most dramatic way of restoring youthful appearance with a laser. The water in skin cells absorbs the laser light, which vaporizers or destroys the cells. Laser resurfacing removes moderate to severe sun damage, leaving remarkably smoother, brighter and firmer skin. By tightening underlying tissues, creating firmer skin, ablative lasers soften the edges of wrinkles and dramatically diminish deep crow's feet or upper lip lines. When lasers are used to resurface the skin, they also can soften the appearance of minor facial scars, such as those produced by acne. Ablative lasers also are used to repair skin that is discolored or has uneven pigment.

What Non-Ablative Lasers Do

These lasers treat skin imperfections by destroying defects caused by tissues beneath the skin, leaving surface layers untouched. Accordingly, there is no wound to the skin surface and healing time is minimal. These lasers are used to make a variety of cosmetic improvements.

Reduce Wrinkles

Non-ablative laser resurfacing causes the collagen layer just beneath the epidermis to gradually thicken, which firms and tones the skin. This helps eliminate finer lines and wrinkles such as those around the eyes, upper lip, cheeks, and forehead. Although you'll need a series of treatments, depending on your skin's

condition, downtime is minimal compared to ablative resurfacing. For this reason, many patients prefer these more frequent, but less aggressive treatments. However, if your skin is heavily damaged, an ablative procedure may be the best option.

Age Spots and Melasma

Depending on the depth and darkness of the melanin pigment that's caused your age spots or pregnancy-related brown splotches, either a non-ablative or ablative laser may be used. Spot treating these areas with a non-ablative laser is a quick and simple procedure; however, in some cases several treatments may be required. Usually, one ablative laser treatment will take care of the spots.

Port-Wine Birthmarks, Spider Veins, Rosacea

One of the remarkable features of non-ablative lasers is their ability to target only cells containing the specific color that causes a skin flaw. For example, problems such as port-wine birth marks, spider veins, and rosacea are vascular, or blood-filled; what they have in common is redness. A laser removes the defects

53

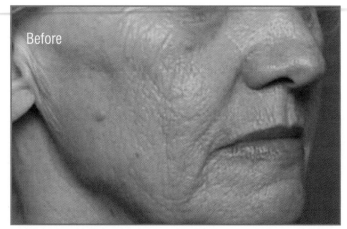

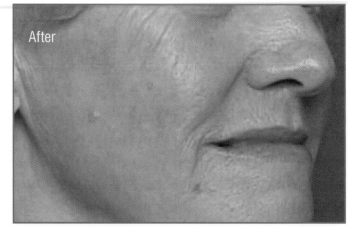

Full-face ablative laser skin resurfacing will treat acne scars and wrinkles.

Healing from ablative laser resurfacing may take several weeks. This patient is shown two months after procedure.

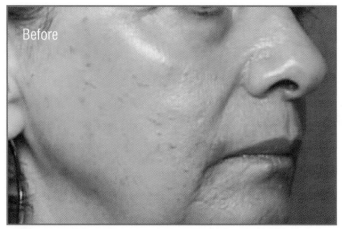

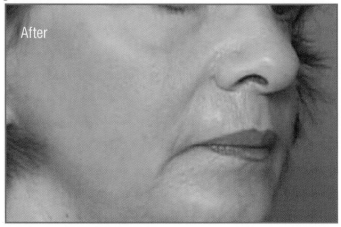

Before full-face laser skin resurfacing. The computerized laser will uniformly remove top layers of skin.

Two months after the laser procedure. These results should last for several years.

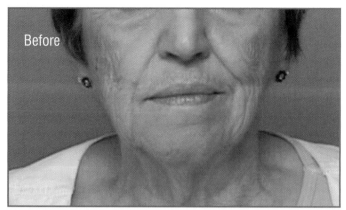

Before full-face laser skin rejuvenation.

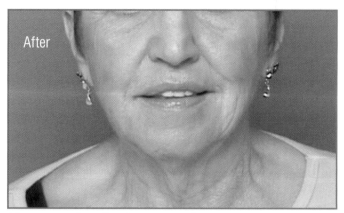

Three months after laser procedure.

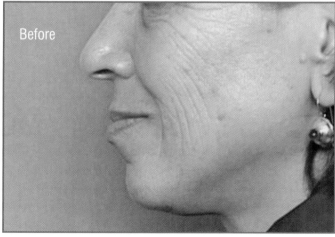

Prior to laser skin resurfacing procedure.

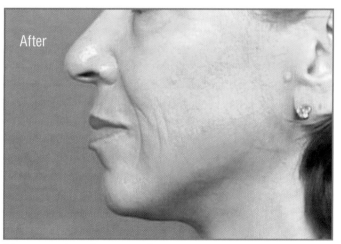

Two months after procedure.

55

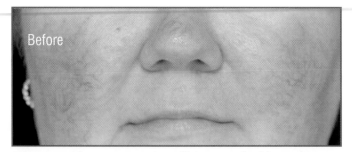

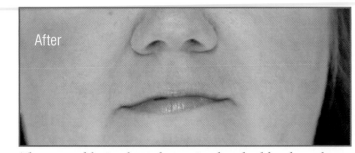

Patient with rosacea, a condition marked by redness on the cheeks, nose, chin, and forehead.

The non-ablative laser beam is absorbed by the color red, collapsing the blood vessels which cause the redness. Surrounding healthy tissue is not affected.

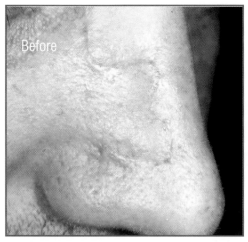

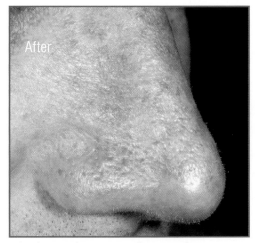

Scar on nose prior to scar revision by ablative laser beam.

The laser eliminates the scar by resurfacing the top layer of skin.

56

by destroying the red hemoglobin, the source of red in the blood. Tiny blood vessels that carry blood to the area are sealed off.

Laser treatment can greatly reduce the reddening common to rosacea. However, laser therapy doesn't cure this condition so you may need periodic touch-ups.

Unwanted Hair

Lasers do a terrific job of removing unwanted hair—with one caveat. They are effective only on dark hair, because the hair-removal laser can target only dark melanin pigment within or near a hair follicle, which helps to destroy the follicle and prevent regrowth. Blonde, red, or gray hair follicles lack this pigment, so laser hair removal isn't effective for them.

Removing Warts and Growths

You can have warts and other small benign growths removed with an ablative laser; in this case it will function like a surgical scalpel. Removal is a simple in-office procedure, so one visit will normally take care of them.

Diminish Scars

Different types of lasers can also reduce the appearance of acne and other scars. As with other laser treatments, the laser is simply passed over the target area. However, depending on the severity of the problem, your doctor may make more than one pass over different spots. The decision to do so is made during the procedure as he or she observes how your skin is responding to the treatment.

A non-ablative laser treatment offers only 10-20 percent improvement, whereas an ablative laser procedure can give 50-60 percent improvement or better.

Non-Ablative Lasers

- Firm and tone the skin
- Remove age spots or melasma
- Remove "spider veins"
- Remove "port wine" birthmarks
- Reduce rosacea reddening
- Remove unwanted hair
- Lessen acne scars, other minor scars
- Remove warts
- Remove tattoos

Lasers Used in Skin Rejuvenation
Ablative Lasers

Carbon dioxide (CO_2)	Renews severely sun-weathered skin by resurfacing the upper layer. Softens the edges of wrinkles and dramatically diminishes deep crow's feet or upper lip lines.
"Superpulsed" CO_2	Renews severely sun-weathered skin by resurfacing the upper layer. Softens the edges of wrinkles, dramatically diminishes deep crow's feet or upper lip lines.
Erbium:YAG	Resurfaces the top layer of skin and tightens underlying tissue. Stimulates the growth of collagen, further diminishing fine lines and wrinkles from mild to moderate sun damage. Improves minor surface scars and splotchy discoloration.

Non-Ablative Lasers

Neodymium	Also known as the Nd:YAG. Laser improves skin firmness and elasticity. Popular version, Cool Touch, uses unique cooling spray that soothes sensitive nerve endings while the laser does its work.
Nd	YAG laser also effective for removing unwanted dark pigment and unwanted hair.
Yellow Light (Pulsed-Dye)	Effectively removes port-wine stains, rosacea, and enlarged blood vessels. Also treats some raised scars and removes red, orange, and yellow tattoo pigments.
Alexandrite and Ruby	Alexandrite laser effective for hair removal in people with darker skin. Ruby laser works best on those with pale skin and dark hair. Both used in tattoo removal. Alexandrite targets black, blue, and green; Ruby removes black, purple, violet, and other dark colors.
Diode	Removes hair in people with fair skin and dark hair. Effective in treating facial spider veins and flat brown spots.

Removing Tattoos

Change your mind about that little daisy tattoo? Lasers can remove most tattoo pigments. For tattoo removal the laser may need to work at a deeper level, so the stinging may be very intense. Because non-ablative lasers work fairly rapidly, however, you won't be uncomfortable for long. Depending on the colors of pigment in a tattoo, separate sessions with different types of lasers may be needed to remove it all.

Are You a Candidate for Laser Treatment?

Laser treatments work best on people with fair skin that is relatively oily, although other skin types have been successfully treated. Only your doctor can determine whether your skin is appropriate for a specific type of laser procedure.

In general, however, non-ablative laser therapy for general skin rejuvenation is most appropriate for younger people with early signs of sun damage. For specific problems such as broken blood vessels or hair removal, age is less significant.

Ablative laser skin resurfacing is a more serious procedure, so your doctor will carefully evaluate your general health and ability to tolerate the removal of a layer of skin. You are not a candidate if you have a current skin infection, have a previous history of severe scarring, or have used Accutane within the last year to two years. Unstable diabetes or autoimmune disorders also rule out laser resurfacing for most people.

Preparing for Laser Treatments

Before laser resurfacing, be sure to fully discuss your medical history with your doctor. It's particularly important to let your doctor know if you have a history of cold sores, herpes, or other viral skin infections, as you will need to take anti-viral medications both before your procedure and during the healing period to prevent a new outbreak. (Actually, all patients are generally treated with prophylactic anti-virals for cold sores.) Also tell your doctor what regular medications and supplements you take, including aspirin, ibuprofen and blood thinners such as Coumadin. (And of course,

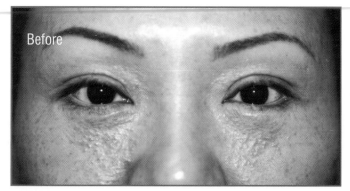

Skin irregularities under the eyes.

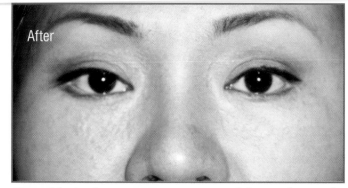

Non-ablative laser treatment removed the top layer of skin, leaving the facial skin refreshed.

you'll want to stop smoking, which impedes skin healing.)

If you have laser hair removal scheduled, you'll need to stop plucking or waxing for four to six weeks in advance. And don't shave for several days before your appointment, as the stubble will help your doctor guide the laser's direction.

If you are undergoing full ablative resurfacing, make arrangements for someone to drive you home because you may feel weak and light-headed from the anesthesia.

To maximize the benefits of any laser treatment, stay out of the sun and be extra vigilant about applying a daily high-SPF sunscreen for two weeks before your procedure as well as forever after!

How Are Ablative Laser Treatments Performed?

Ablative laser skin resurfacing is one of the more aggressive forms of skin rejuvenation. The procedure must be performed in an operating room or surgical suite. Although this is not an invasive surgical procedure, you will be hooked up to an EKG, a heart monitor, and a blood pressure cuff. Because anesthetics used can stimulate the heart, routine monitoring is required. You'll also wear a small device, a pulse oximeter, on your index finger to monitor your blood oxygen level.

To guard against infection, your skin will be cleansed with disinfectant, and you'll be covered with sterile drapes. You'll also be wearing special goggles to protect your eyes from the laser light.

Depending on the procedure, your doctor may apply a topical anesthetic. More often, ablative resurfacing requires either an injected nerve block or twilight sedation, which is given through an IV. When extensive work is needed, general anesthesia will usually be recommended.

As the treatment starts, the doctor will use an instrument about the size of a pencil to pass the laser beam over your skin, removing the epidermis and part of the upper dermis. Because the laser is fully computerized, your doctor can precisely control the amount of energy in the beam, the density of the light, and the length of time it stays on your skin. Depending on your skin's condition and the areas to be treated, the procedure will take from thirty minutes to over an hour. Some parts of the face may require a second pass; your doctor

will carefully avoid letting the laser's light penetrate too deeply. In many cases, as doctors treat the skin surface, they also see the skin firming up as the laser is passed across the face.

After your ablative resurfacing is done, your face will be wrapped in either an antibiotic-soaked gauze bandage or a mask-like dressing that resembles plastic wrap. You'll wear these important dressings several days because they help your skin retain moisture and prevent exposure to the air, which might encourage scabs to form and cause scarring. You'll rest in a recovery area for a few hours until any lingering light-headedness from the sedation or anesthesia has worn off. Then you'll need a friend or relative to drive you home. In the first few days, you'll need to return to the doctor's office several times for dressing changes.

Full recovery from ablative resurfacing is lengthy and can take two to six weeks. Women should usually wait about two weeks before they apply makeup and return to work. Men usually grow their beards for two to three weeks which helps camouflage their pink skin. For both sexes, the pinkness gradually fades

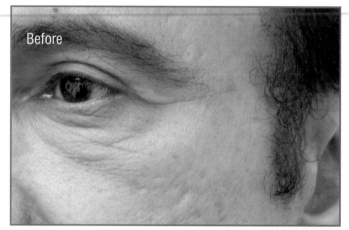

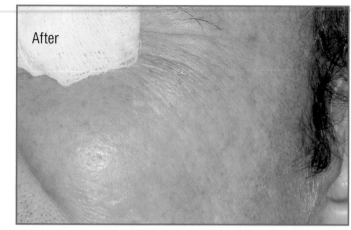

Shallow acne scars. Non-ablative laser will stimulate collagen growth, filling in the scars. Surface skin will not be injured.

After laser treatment. Results will improve further during the next several months.

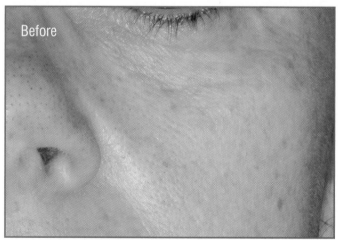

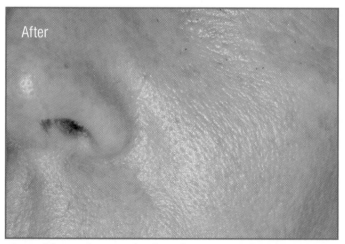

Patient wishes to diminish nasolabial fold and improve skin tone.

Non-ablative laser refreshes skin, erases fine lines, and softens nasolabial folds.

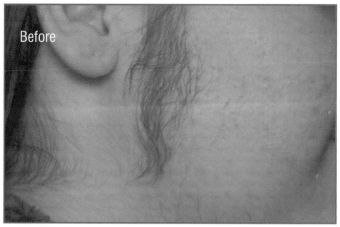

Laser hair removal. For good results, hair must be darker than surrounding skin.

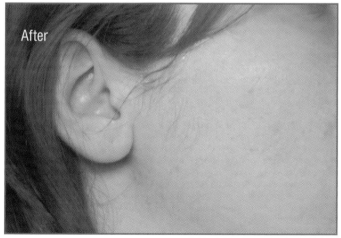

To permanently remove hair, several laser treatments are usually required.

over the next two to three months. How quickly it does so is dependent on the regimen the physician uses with the patient (skin care products both pre- and post-laser) and how closely the patient follows it. Recovery time frames vary widely with the individual.

How Are Non-Ablative Laser Treatments Performed?

These procedures can be done in the doctor's office. You'll lie on a table or recline in a dental-style chair, with a simple gown or medical smock over your clothing. You'll wear protective eye goggles.

Your need for any anesthetic will vary depending on the complexity of your skin problem and your pain tolerance. A fairly superficial age spot, for example, will normally produce brief strong stinging but nothing intense enough to require a numbing cream. If you are having a blood vessel or deep pigment area corrected, you may require either an injection of lidocaine or a topical cream, which should numb the area in about twenty minutes. Ask your doctor what kind of pain relief would be most appropriate for you.

After your skin is cleansed, your doctor will pass the laser's hand piece over the affected area on your face. You may occasionally hear a sharp "pop." This noise is simply the sound of the laser fizzling a hair within a follicle. These follicles are present in many parts of your skin, even where you have only light, barely visible facial hairs.

These procedures usually take about fifteen minutes. Afterward, you may be given a cold gel pack to place over your face for a few minutes afterward to cool any residual burning you may feel.

Hair Removal

You'll usually be offered a topical anesthetic cream for hair removal, because this procedure often involves larger target areas, such as the upper lip, chin, cheeks, or neck. Your skin will be numb after twenty to thirty minutes after the cream is applied.

After laser hair removal, mild swelling and redness around the follicles are normal, but these usually disappear within a few hours. Occasionally, red bumps as distinct as mosquito bites may appear for a few days. This

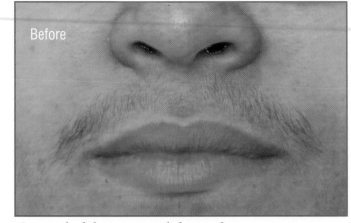

Coarse dark hair responds best to laser treatment.

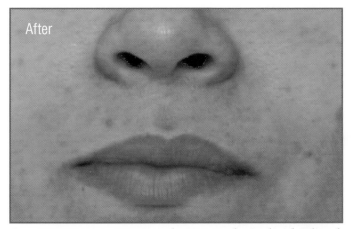

Laser treatment to remove hair must be individualized. Some people get lasting results from one procedure. Others require more treatments.

reaction tends to be more severe on the legs or in the bikini area.

It takes a series of at least three treatments to remove unwanted hair, because hair grows in cycles. Some follicles are dormant, while others are actively producing a hair; the laser can destroy only the follicles that are active at the time of your treatment.

How Will I Look?

After Ablative Laser Resurfacing

Immediately afterward, your face will look as though you've had a major sunburn. It will be swollen for about three days. Your skin will be raw and may "weep." As mentioned, your face will be covered with antibiotic ointments or light bandages for several days.

After the bandages and ointments are gone, you'll see much softer, pinker, and smoother skin. Most lines and wrinkles will be radically reduced if not eliminated entirely, along with roughness and pigmentation spots. During the next several months, the changes generated by new collagen formation will slowly appear. Your skin will appear firmer and tighter, in many cases dramatically so.

After Non-Ablative Laser Treatment

If you've had a blood vessel or a pigmented area such as an age spot or tattoo removed, the skin will immediately turn white and then change to a reddish-purple color about five to ten minutes after the treatment. Mild swelling is possible, but normally not enough to be noticeable to anyone else. Your skin color will gradually return to normal over a one- to two-week period. (You can disguise it with makeup in the meantime.)

Follow-Up Care

After Ablative Skin Resurfacing

You'll be visiting your doctor again a few days to a week after your procedure to have the dressings removed, and you'll be given specific instructions for your follow-up care. Pain is generally minimal and most patients use narcotics for one day, if at all. To further the healing process, you will want to take the following steps:

- Sleep on two pillows for a week or two to reduce swelling.
- Follow the detailed instructions from your doctor on how to apply the

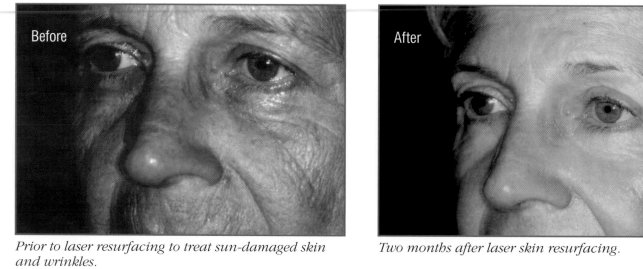

Prior to laser resurfacing to treat sun-damaged skin and wrinkles.

Two months after laser skin resurfacing.

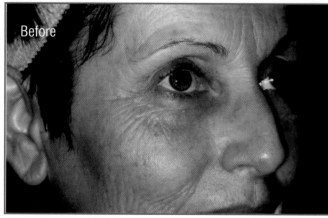

Prior to laser treatment.

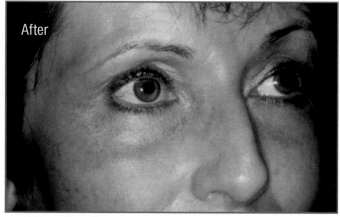

Seven weeks after laser skin resurfacing.

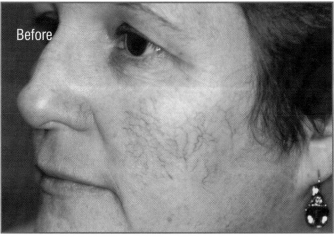

Spider veins on the cheeks.

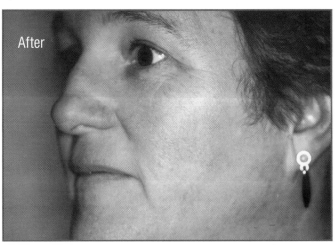

Laser beam has destroyed the red cells in spider veins without damaging healthy cells.

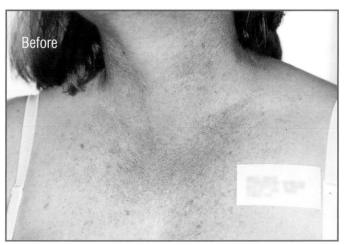

Sun damage to decolletage.

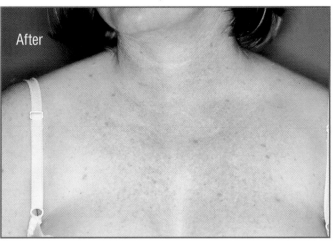

Renewed skin, several weeks after laser skin resurfacing.

67

ointments and replace the protective dressings.

- Wash your face several times a day with a gentle warm-water spray and the soap your doctor provides.

- Take any other medications, antibiotics or anti-viral medications, your doctor has prescribed for you.

- Become a sunscreen zealot—safeguard your new skin with generous daily applications of a high-quality, high-SPF sunscreen.

Depending on the depth of your treatment, your healing time may vary from one to several weeks. You may be able to return to work wearing makeup after only one week.

After Non-Ablative Laser Treatments

In most cases, non-ablative laser sessions require minimal follow-up. The basics include not picking or scratching at the skin while any discoloration remains, and faithfully using a high-SPF sunblock. If you choose to wear makeup afterward, ask your doctor what kind is appropriate, and apply and remove it very gently.

How Long Will Results Last?

The length of time any laser treatment lasts varies. You can't stop the march of time, of course, but you can slow it to a crawl if you avoid further sun damage, eat a nutritious diet, don't smoke or drink to excess, and follow a healthy skin-care regimen. Other predictions depend on the condition of your skin when you sought laser therapy and the nature and severity of the problem you had corrected.

Ablative Laser Resurfacing

With proper skin care and sun protection, the results of a complete resurfacing in most cases will last a minimum of five years, and for many people even eight or ten years. As the aging process continues, you will see gradual changes appear. It is unusual to repeat a complete ablative resurfacing, but throughout the years, your doctor can offer a variety of complementary treatments to prolong the renewed appearance of your skin.

Non-Ablative Laser Treatments

Although it often takes a series of six to ten non-ablative treatments to achieve the best results, once a vascular or pigment problem is corrected or a tattoo is removed, the result is permanent. However, if your aim was simply to counteract overall mild sun damage, you may decide on an additional series of treatments after several years to treat continuing sun damage and aging. For ongoing permanent hair removal, you may need touch-up sessions a few years later, as new hair follicles continue to develop.

Potential Risks

Ablative laser resurfacing, because it exposes a raw new layer, introduces the same risk of infection as any technique that removes a significant depth of skin. Proper follow-up care can protect you from the possibility of infection. If there is undiagnosed herpes simplex virus (HSV) present in the skin, it may be activated by the laser and produce scarring.

Non-ablative laser treatments are considered extremely safe. However, as with any procedure, scarring can occur in some individuals. If you are in the care of an experienced physician, the risk is very small. Proper screening to be sure you do not have a history of severe scarring is important. Rarely, white spots or other pigmentation problems can appear after laser treatments, particularly in people with dark or olive-toned skin.

Questions to Ask Your Doctor

- Do I have any condition that would make me a poor candidate for laser treatment?
- If I have a series of non-ablative laser treatments, how far apart should they be?
- How many initial treatments would you recommend for me?

- Is laser therapy likely to achieve the improvement I'm looking for?
- If not, what other types of treatment would you suggest?
- Should I stop taking my usual medications or supplements?

Six

Microdermabrasion

Microdermabrasion

Remember skinning your knees and shins when you were little? Those minor injuries, which scraped away the top layer of skin, are called *abrasions.* What you may remember too is that once the abrasion healed and the scabs fell away, the new skin underneath was softer, smoother, and pinker than the surrounding skin.

In principle, abrasion can do the same thing for aging facial skin. Used in a carefully controlled manner to rub away a weathered surface, abrading the skin allows tender new skin to appear. To rejuvenate skin, two types of abrasion are used: traditional dermabrasion and microdermabrasion. Both treatments basically involve "sanding" the skin surface to a smoother finish, but at different depths. The difference between them is really just a matter of degree.

With *dermabrasion,* a rotating wire brush or similar surgical tool is used to literally "sand" off the entire top layer of your skin, the epidermis. In skilled hands, dermabrasion is very effective for severely sun-damaged and deeply wrinkled areas of skin. It does involve considerable bleeding, however, and several weeks of recovery time.

Microdermabrasion is dermabrasion's gentler cousin. Often called a "power peel" or "French peel," the procedure was popular in Europe for nearly a decade before coming to the United States in the late 1990s. Microdermabrasion also "sands" facial skin to new smoothness, but with a gentle stream of microscopic crystals rather than a brush. It's a quick, virtually painless, and very popular method for renewing tired-looking skin. Microdermabrasion doesn't create a dramatically new skin layer as dermabrasion does, but with repeated treatments, it can make a remarkable difference in creating a more youthful face.

What Microdermabrasion Does

Microdermabrasion removes the topmost layer of skin, mostly composed of dead skin cells and pore-clogging debris, along with a very small amount of the next skin layer, the dermis. A microdermabrasion treatment freshens and exfoliates skin, repairing minor sun damage and smoothing dry areas. Because debris and dead cells are removed, whiteheads and blackheads are also diminished. Microdermabrasion can be effective in helping to control acne, too. It creates a healthier environment where new skin cells can regenerate naturally.

There is virtually no trauma involved with microdermabrasion and, likewise, because there is no "wound" to the skin, there's no downtime. Many people schedule treatments during a lunch hour and go right back to work with a fresh new glow. The maximum benefits of microdermabrasion, such as reducing the

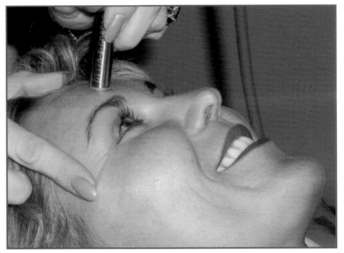

Microdermabrasion gently exfoliates the top layer of the skin with sterile crystals, and simultaneously vacuums the dead skin cells.

appearance of fine lines, age spots, uneven skin tone, shallow acne scars, and moderate sun damage, appear not after one treatment, but after a series of treatments. The fragile skin of the neck, which often cannot tolerate stronger methods, can usually be safely smoothed with microdermabrasion. For example, if the neck and upper chest have sustained sun damage, these areas are also treated, blending the skin tone with that of the face.

Are You a Candidate for Microdermabrasion?

Because it's such a gentle procedure, almost anyone can enjoy the refreshing exfoliation of microdermabrasion. Virtually all skin types can benefit. Microdermabrasion is particularly useful for people who have such busy schedules that they can't take the time to recover from more powerful resurfacing treatments. It's important to know, however, that microdermabrasion will not "lift" sagging skin or re-contour the shape of the face.

Unless you have severely inflamed acne, rosacea, warts, or undiagnosed skin lesions of any kind, you are likely an excellent candidate for microdermabrasion. If you have had recent outbreaks of the herpes virus that causes cold sores, your doctor may prescribe a ten-day course of antiviral medication before you have a microdermabrasion treatment. As stated earlier, the presence of an active cold sore could cause the viral infection to spread as a result of the procedure. If you've had a recent sunburn or windburn, you'll need to wait until your skin has recovered.

The only major medical conditions that rule out microdermabrasion are unstable diabetes and autoimmune disorders. These conditions may impair healing.

After microdermabrasion, my skin is softer and brighter. It cleans out the pores and shrinks them. My face is only slightly pinker after the procedure, and I go right back to work.

Jan, 47

Preparing for Microdermabrasion

Don't use any scrubs, lotions, loofahs, astringent masques, or similar exfoliating products on your skin for at least a week before your appointment. You might want to wear less makeup than usual that day, as your face will need to be cleansed once you're at the doctor's office.

How Is Microdermabrasion Performed?

The procedure is quite simple—some people even find it relaxing. You'll be sitting comfortably, and no anesthesia is required. The "sand" used during microdermabrasion is much finer than grains of real sand. The primary exfoliating particles are aluminum oxide crystals, but in some cases other tiny particles are used, made of substances such as baking soda, salt, or corn cobs (ground to an extremely fine consistency).

First, a cleansing toner is applied all over your face to remove every trace of makeup or oil. Then your doctor uses a special "wand" that looks something like a dentist's drill to pass a steady stream of the fine abrasive particles over your skin, working over one small area at a time. As the wand delivers the crystals, it also works as a vacuum—removing dead cells, debris, and a tiny amount of surface skin.

The process lasts about twenty to thirty minutes, depending on the depth of the treatment. In areas that are especially dry or may need a little extra abrasion, your doctor can adjust the crystals' flow for a stronger effect.

You will feel a tingle from the stream of particles, but most people describe no pain, and some even find it pleasant. The exception is that the area around the eyes may sting a little, because your skin is thinner and more sensitive there. But again, the sensation is not strong enough to require any kind of anesthetic—your skin may feel a little hot, but that's about the extent of it. In a short time, the procedure's done. To finish the process, a cotton ball with a soothing toner will be passed over your face, followed by a rehydrating cream.

How Will I Look?

Immediately after a microdermabrasion, your skin will turn pink for a few hours, and it may feel a little dry and flaky over the next day or two. This is normal and, in fact, the mild peeling is one of the benefits of the treatment. Right away, you'll detect more softness and smoothness, and you may notice that makeup goes on much more easily.

> *I love microdermabrasion. It literally vacuums my face. My skin glows. I wear less makeup now than ever in my life.*
> Susan, 48

If you decide to have a series of treatments, then over time you'll notice greater changes in the look of your skin—more even skin tone and a much smoother surface texture. Very fine lines and mild age spots will be diminished or will disappear.

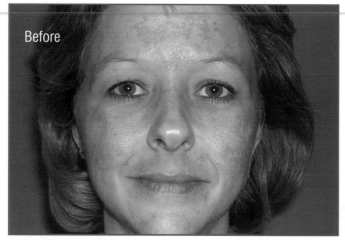

Before

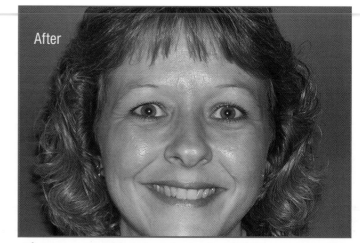

After

Mottled pigmentation and rough skin texture.

After seven weekly microdermabrasion treatments, skin is smoother and skin tone is even.

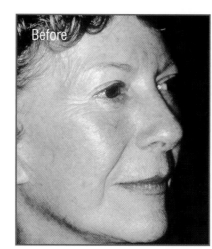

Before

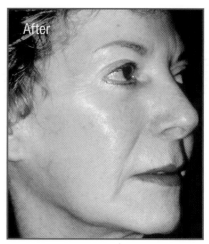

After

Skin tone is uneven and crow's feet are distinct.

Six weeks later, after weekly treatments, skin tone is even and crow's feet are softened.

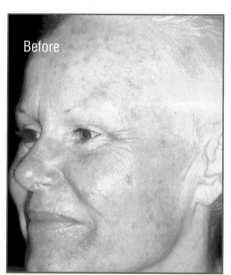

Before

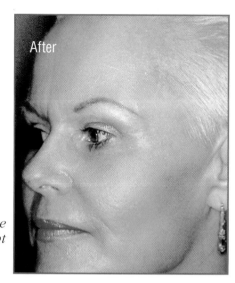

After

Skin is sun-damaged and fine lines are visible.

Seven weeks later, fine lines are diminished and renewed skin surface shows even with light makeup.

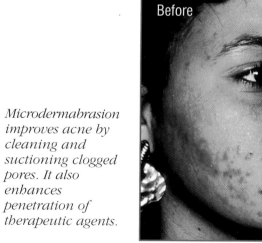

Before

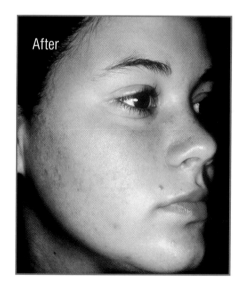

After

Microdermabrasion improves acne by cleaning and suctioning clogged pores. It also enhances penetration of therapeutic agents.

After eight weekly microdermabrasion treatments.

Microdermabrasion Improves:

- Acne
- Sun damage
- Hyperpigmentation
- Fine lines
- Mild scarring
- Keratosis
- Overall skin texture

Follow-Up Care

In the majority of cases, there's no significant aftercare required. Microdermabrasion treatments do remove just enough surface skin to make it more vulnerable to the sun, so after treatment you'll want to apply a good quality, high-SPF sunblock. Your doctor may also advise you to avoid using strong scrubs or exfoliating lotions at home, since microdermabrasion does a better and more controlled job.

How Long Will Results Last?

Just one microdermabrasion treatment can invigorate your face. Until a new layer of the stratum corneum develops, you'll enjoy the refreshed appearance of your skin. To maintain or deepen the procedure's benefits, however, most doctors suggest a series of treatments. The intervals recommended will vary according to the condition of your skin and your individual needs, but in general, a series of three to six weekly treatments is the best way to start. After that, the benefits of microdermabrasion can usually be maintained with follow-up treatments at three- to six-month intervals.

Potential Risks

Overall, microdermabrasion is one of the least painful and least risky skin resurfacing techniques. There are very few risks with microdermabrasion, other than a slight possibility of pigmentation change. This is likely to happen only if a person with dark skin receives a treatment in which the stream of crystals is applied too forcefully. This is a very unusual occurrence, however.

If crystals become embedded in the pores of a person with severe acne, a skin infection could result. However, this problem is easily prevented by proper screening of patients with acne.

Questions to Ask Your Doctor

- Do I have any conditions that would make me a poor candidate for microdermabrasion?

- If I have a series of treatments, how far apart should they be?

- How many initial treatments would you recommend for me?

- Is microdermabrasion sufficient to achieve the improvement I'm looking for?

- If not, what other types of treatment would you suggest?

- Should I stop taking my usual medications or supplements?

Seven

Fillers: Injections and Implants

Fillers: Injections and Implants

In recent years, wrinkle filling has become one of the most sought-after facial rejuvenation procedures. Perhaps the filler you're most familiar with is *collagen*, which is delivered by injection. However, a variety of other fillers are also available, and more are hitting the market.

You may have thought that fillers could remove only very fine lines, not the deeper wrinkles and folds. Not so! Today there are many filling techniques for plumping up the skin and smoothing even the deepest wrinkles.

What Fillers Do

Fillers, often referred to as *soft-tissue fillers*, fill in grooves or creases, smoothing them and blending them into the rest of your skin. Fillers are also used in simple procedures to augment the chin and to fill in deep creases in the cheeks, restoring the rounded contour of the cheekbones. Fillers come in two forms: filler injections and filler implants. Filler injections are typically used for nasolabial folds, forehead lines, crow's feet, smile lines, frown lines, and wrinkles around the lips. Filler implants are frequently used to fill creases in the cheeks or to strengthen the chin or firm the jawline.

Just as your face is unique, so are the patterns of your wrinkles. Accordingly, there's no one-filler-fits-all solution. After a careful examination of your face, your doctor will help you make the determination of which types of fillers or combinations of fillers are the best choice for you.

Temporary Fillers

Fillers are temporary when the material used is eventually reabsorbed by the body.

Temporary injectables can also provide an ideal way to try out a wrinkle-filling or tissue-lifting technique before considering a more permanent method. These filler injections are popular because they are quick and involve virtually no downtime.

Collagen

Collagen injections are effective for the correction of smile or frown lines, nasolabial folds, and delicate lines at the corners of the eyes. Collagen is also used to fill lines around the mouth, adding definition to the lips. And, it is effective for filling acne scars. Collagen is a natural protein, a substance that forms part of the supporting structure under the skin. However, our own supplies of collagen naturally diminish with age. Using collagen for cosmetic purposes was first introduced in the United States more than twenty years ago. During that time, most collagen fillers were derived from purified bovine (cow) collagen.

In March 2003, the FDA approved the first human-based collagen products, made from natural dermal tissue grown under controlled laboratory conditions. This is the same tissue-engineering technology that has been

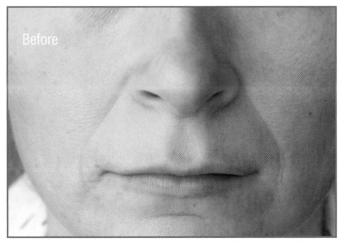

Before injections of human-based collagen to soften nasolabial folds.

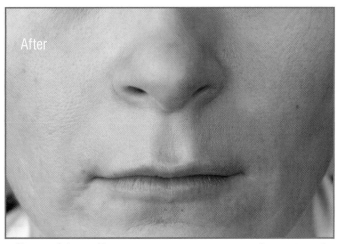

Effects of the collagen injections are immediate. Results will last for several months.

successfully used for years to create living tissues for the treatment of burns and other skin wounds. Marketed as *CosmoDerm*™ and *CosmoPlast,*™ these products eliminate the concern over allergic reactions to bovine collagen.

Unlike other dermal fillers, both forms of collagen contain an anesthetic for patient comfort. Treatment results are immediate and last from three to six months.

Hyaluronic Acid

Our bodies produce *hyaluronic acid,* a structural part of the skin that creates volume and shape and acts as a lubricant and shock absorber. But our natural supplies shrink with age. A new soft-tissue filler is making its way onto the market. You may have heard it referred to by the brand names *Restylane* and *Perlane.* Even though it is synthetic, it is very similar to natural hyaluronic acid.

First popularized in Europe, South America, and Canada, the gel-like substance stimulates one's own natural skin cells to "float" upward to the surface. As a result, creases and grooves are filled in more naturally. This makes these injections particularly useful for treating

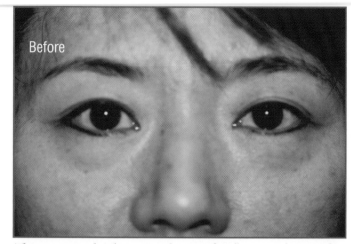

This woman had an autologous fat (her own) transfer to her lower eye lids.

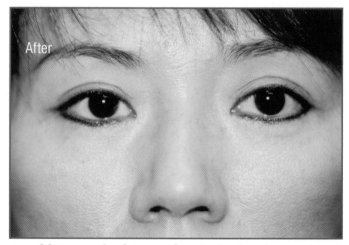

In addition to the fat transfer, she had a chemical peel to even her skin tone.

Temporary Injectables

	HYALURONIC ACID	BOTULINUM TOXIN	FAT INJECTIONS	COLLAGEN	
Trade Name	Restylane, Perlane, and Restylane Fine Lines	Botox and Myoblo	Fat Injection	Zyderm and Zyplast	CosmoDerm and CosmoPlast
What It Is	A substance found in all living organisms	Botulinum toxin type A, produced by *Clostridia Botulinum* bacteria	Fat transfer from one part of the body to another	Natural substances derived from purified bovine (cow) collagen	Human collagen developed in a laboratory
How It Works	For volume and shaping	Temporarily relaxes the muscle	Adds volume	Adds volume	Adds volume
Injection Areas	Nasolabial folds, forehead wrinkles, smile lines, and lips	Forehead, frown lines, crow's feet, and vertical neck bands	Nasolabial folds, frown lines, crow's feet, lips, and facial recontouring	Nasolabial folds, frown lines, crow's feet, and lips	Nasolabial folds, frown lines, crow's feet, and lips
Results	Up to 12 months	Up to 6 months	Highly variable: months to years	Up to 6 months	Up to 6 months
U.S. Availability	No (FDA approval pending for cosmetic use)	Yes	Yes	Yes	Yes
Back To Work	No downtime	No downtime	Minor: 1-4 days Extensive: 7-14 days	No downtime	No downtime
Possible Reactions	Swelling, redness, and tenderness	Bruising, redness, droopy eyelid, headache, and flu like symptoms	Swelling, bruising, and lumpiness	Slight bruising and allergic reactions	Slight bruising and allergic reactions
Other Considerations	None identified at this time	None identified at this time	Requires a donor site (for example, abdomen, buttocks or thighs)	Requires a skin test for allergic reaction and at least one month wait	No pre-treatment skin test required

Courtesy American Society for Aesthetic Plastic Surgery

nasolabial folds, lip lines, smile lines, and drooping corners of the mouth. It is also used to fill fine to moderate wrinkles as well as scars. The results last for about twelve months.

Autologous Fat

Injections of your own autologous body fat can be used to reduce deeper facial wrinkles or fill in the hollows that have gradually appeared. These fat deposits can be drawn from such areas as the buttocks, thighs, or abdomen and are quickly processed into injectable form in the doctor's office. Sometimes the fat is extracted during a mini-liposuction procedure or is taken from a simple incision in an area such as the back of the knee. Because this is your body's own tissue, there is no risk of allergy or rejection. In some cases, the results last only a month or two; in others, they last years, depending on how soon your body reabsorbs the fat.

If a patient is tentative about having a filler treatment, I will suggest temporary filler. Then, if patient is happy with the results, I will recommend a longer-acting filler or permanent implant.

Dr. Jon Mendelsohn
Facial Plastic Surgeon

Fascia Lata

Another treatment derived from your own or donor tissue, this filler consists of tiny pieces of the *fascia lata*, the firm, white collagen-rich layer that covers the muscles, just underneath body fat. Fascia is commonly harvested from the muscle above the ear through a small incision above the hairline. Originally small pieces were used only in surgery to fill deep scars, but it is now possible to process fascia into an injectable used to augment lips and smooth wrinkles. Like autologous fat, fascia lata is sometimes used as an alternative for people who show an allergic response to bovine collagen. Results should last three to six months.

Permanent Fillers

Depending on which type you choose, permanent fillers can give results ranging from semipermanent to "lasting as long as you do." Some of the newest permanent fillers are liquid blends of natural materials and tiny particles of vinyl or polymer. Other permanent fillers are solid or mesh-like implants, inserted through tiny incisions.

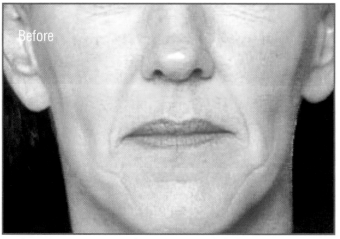

Before the insertion of implants to fill the nasolabial folds.

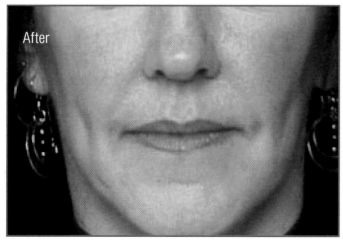

After the insertion of two soft strands of implant material. The results are permanent.

Hybrids

One of the newer filler products in the consumer market is known as a hybrid filler—it is considered permanent. Marketed under the brand name *Artefill*, it is a blend of microscopically tiny plastic beads and collagen. The body absorbs the collagen in a few months, but the permanent tiny beads stimulate the production of the body's own collagen. The new collagen encapsulates the beads, making the filler permanent. The result: skin volume is boosted. The hybrid filler may be used for wrinkles, deep nasolabial folds, frown lines, and acne scars.

Bio-Implants

These implants, once inserted under the skin, actually function like a scaffold to be slowly filled in by your body's own collagen. Although they are manufactured, they are produced from skin, fascia, or collagen harvested from donors and processed in a laboratory in such a way that it becomes biologically "generic." Normally, your body will accept this natural, treated tissue as its own. Bio-implants are injected within a liquid base, rather than inserted through an incision.

87

Bio-implants are often effective for wrinkles, deep folds, frown lines between the brows, lip augmentation, and filling in acne scars.

Synthetic Implants

These solid, permanent implants are made from a polymer similar to Gore-Tex, the material used to make boots and raincoats. However, the implant material is a medical grade. The polymer is firm but feels flexible. The implants come in various forms and shapes, including sheets, mesh-like strips, oval pieces, and round, tubular threads. Synthetic implants are used for filling nasolabial folds and for lip augmentation.

Silicone

One well-known though controversial permanent filler treatment is silicone. Liquid silicone has been offered for years in micro-droplet injection form by some physicians who believe that, used appropriately, it is safe and effective. However, debate over the safety of silicone continues in the medical community. Many doctors avoid silicone because of its history of causing problems in

some patients, including migration or shifting of the silicone, infection, and hardening.

Are You a Candidate for Fillers?

If you have persistent wrinkles that have not responded to more superficial measures, you may be an excellent candidate for a filler treatment. You may also be a candidate if, along with maturity, aging has brought you a "hollowed" look. Other people decide to investigate these options after losing a great deal of weight, which sometimes causes faces to appear not just thinner, but gaunt, particularly in the cheeks. Or, perhaps you have a weak or recessive chin, which can add to early jowling and makes one's nose appear larger in profile.

Because there are so many ways to fill different types of wrinkles and reshape facial contours, you and your physician will want to review the options together and select the treatments that will work best for you. It is a very customized process, and often a combination of different types of fillers will produce the best results.

If you have a history of allergy to meat or other bovine products, or severe allergies in

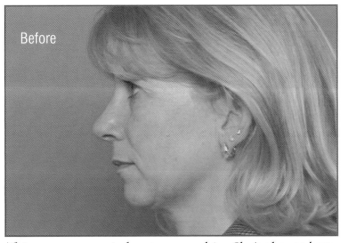

This woman wanted a stronger chin. She's shown here prior to the insertion of a rubber-like chin implant.

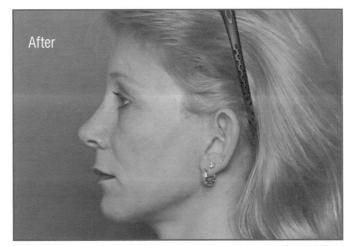

After the insertion of the permanent chin implant. The procedure was performed in about fifteen minutes under local anesthetic.

general, you may not be a good candidate for bovine collagen. (About one in one hundred people tests positive for bovine allergy.) However, you will more likely be a candidate for the newer human-based collagen. Any clotting disorders or allergies to local anesthesia may also mean that implants are not a good choice for you.

Preparing for a Filler Procedure

For virtually all the injectable fillers, no advance preparation is needed. The exception is a simple skin test to rule out the possibility of an allergic reaction to bovine collagen. After a tiny amount of the solution is injected in a location elsewhere on your body, such as the arm, you'll need to watch the area closely for four weeks for signs of an allergic response, such as severe itching, swelling, or redness.

Most reactions occur within three days, but the four-week window is necessary, because a reaction could occur anytime during this period. However, if your doctor recommends human-based collagen, you won't need a pre-treatment skin test.

Before an implant procedure, your doctor will let you know whether you need to stop taking certain medications. Taking aspirin and other blood-thinning drugs or supplements is generally not advisable before any incision, although the incisions for facial implants are so tiny that this caution may be unnecessary. This will depend on your individual health history, which you'll discuss with your doctor. And of course, if you haven't already, stop smoking! Smoking can create new wrinkles and squint lines and undo the benefits of your treatment.

> *Having a weak chin always bothered me. I had no idea getting a chin implant was such a simple procedure. I had it done over my lunch hour.*
>
> Lou, 26

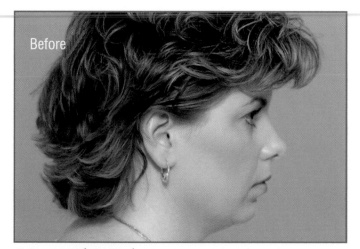

Prior to a chin implant.

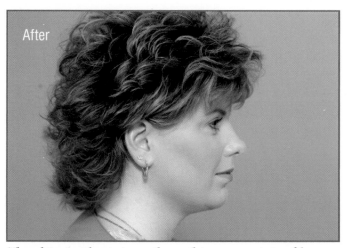

The chin implant strengthens this woman's profile.

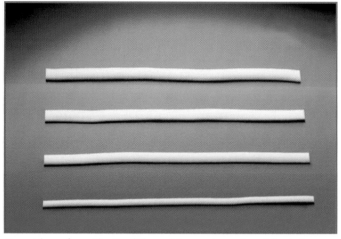

Samples of synthetic fillers. These strands of facial implant material are used to fill nasolabial folds and to augment lips.

How Are Fillers Injected or Implanted?

Filler Injections

Once you and your doctor have decided where you would like to have fillers injected, the areas are cleaned with alcohol. Most fillers do not require a topical anesthetic—they sting only as much as any shot. However, *lidocaine*, a local anesthetic, is normally included in the syringe, so the discomfort won't last long.

Exceptions: if you are receiving a series of collagen injections, you will likely experience discomfort because it's a fairly thick liquid. After each bit of collagen is injected, the doctor or nurse rapidly rubs the area for a few seconds to distribute the collagen evenly, which will also be uncomfortable. Most patients tolerate hyaluronic acid injections quite well and often do not require a local anesthetic.

If you have concerns about pain, ask your doctor about an anesthetic. If your chosen filler liquid is suitable for smaller needles, it may be possible to receive micro-injections. In addition to local anesthetics such as lidocaine, a *nerve block anesthetic* is also an option in some cases. A nerve block is a deeper, more targeted injection of anesthetic into tissue containing sensory nerves in areas around the lips.

Filler Implants

Most implants used for wrinkles are produced in strips or threads, so each piece of material has two ends and is "threaded" through the area of tissue being filled. After the location for each incision is disinfected, a local anesthetic will be injected. Once the skin is numb, the doctor will make a tiny incision at each end of the crease or wrinkle. Then, with a special threading device, the implant material is pulled from one incision through to the other incision. Next, the ends are trimmed and a single, hair-thin stitch is placed at each end to hold the implant in place while the incisions heal. In some cases, a kind of suture is used that will simply fall out on its own. Otherwise, your doctor will need to remove the stitches in a few days.

The incisions' locations will vary, of course, with the location of the wrinkle or groove being filled. Basically, however, incisions are hidden at the top and bottom of the line or fold being treated.

Other solid implants are shaped like wedges or cookies. These implants—the type used for filling out "sunken" cheeks—are trimmed to fit the precise area of your face. These implants are highly flexible and can be placed under the skin through very small incisions. In many cases, one incision can be placed inside the cheek or mouth, so only one is made on the outside of the face. Your physician may attempt to make the tiny incision in a spot such as a dimple, where it

would be hidden. Regardless of where the incision to anchor the other end of the implant is placed, there is no noticeable scar, because the incision is so tiny.

For a chin implant, a local anesthetic is also used. A tiny incision is made either between the inner lower lip and the teeth or under the chin, where it is not noticeable. After the custom implant is inserted, the incision is closed with sutures that dissolve is several days. The procedure takes about fifteen minutes, and a patient can return to work. The result is permanent and the chin feels natural to patients.

How Will I Look?

After a Filler Injection

One of the reasons injection fillers are so popular is that the results are virtually instantaneous. The wrinkle or "sunken" area will be softened and less pronounced, and your face will be subtly redefined. For a few days, you may have a little temporary swelling or puffiness, so the result you first see in the mirror will improve once the swelling resolves. Some short-term redness is possible, too.

After a Filler Implant

A synthetic implant can reshape your face more distinctly than an injection. Swelling will usually be more pronounced with implants than with injections, but will be gone in a few days. Temporary bruising often appears on the skin above where an implant is placed, but this can be covered by makeup.

The improvement is seen immediately; however, the final, filled-in effect of your implants is normally apparent after about three months, when your own tissue growth has had time to make its contribution, too. You will notice that the treated areas of your face look firmer, with more defined contours. Where once there was a depression or deep groove, a smoother, younger-looking surface has appeared.

After a chin implant procedure, you'll have an immediate improvement to your profile. The implant will also add balance to the frontal view of your face. There may or may not be slight bruising afterwards.

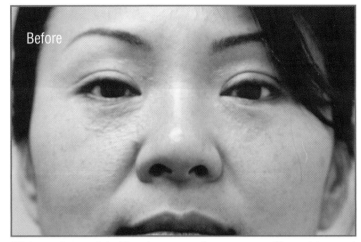

This patient wished to improve the texture of her skin and diminish the creases in her nasolabial folds.

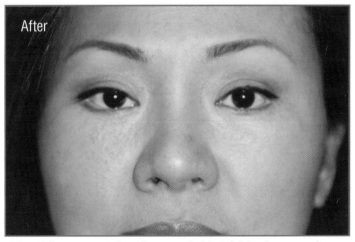

After filler material to the nasolabial folds, fat transfer to the lower eyelids, and laser skin resurfacing.

93

Follow-Up Care

Your doctor will give you detailed instructions on how to care for your skin after your treatment. Because filler options vary so widely, the follow-up care varies too. For most injections, you'll simply need to keep your face clean of cosmetics for a day. If any swelling is bothering you, you might want to apply a simple cold pack, wrapped in a towel, for fifteen minutes every hour or two.

For some procedures, such as fat injections or implants, it will also be important to avoid making animated facial expressions. This allows the material to "settle" into the tissues of your face and allows your body's own tissue regrowth to begin relatively undisturbed. Likewise, too much motion might be uncomfortable. (Laughing for hours the same evening, for example, might leave you with an aching face.) You won't need to walk around with a frozen expression, but try to avoid a great deal of exaggerated facial motions such as huge yawning or cheering at a sports event. Periodic ice packs are often recommended for the first twenty-four to forty-eight hours.

How Long Will Results Last?

As mentioned throughout this chapter, the results of temporary injectable wrinkle fillers can last anywhere from three months to a year. Some of the newer soft-tissue fillers may last up to two years. These results vary from person to person, depending on how your own body responds to the substance. How long your results last largely depends on the depth of the area treated, how much material is injected, and how much of your own collagen and tissue repair your body produces. Because of these variables, your best guide will be what you observe in the mirror.

Permanent implant fillers are just that. Most of them will last longer than you do, unless for some reason you decide to have them removed. Occasionally, individuals request removal because they are not happy with how an implant looks, or are unusually sensitive to its "feel." More often, people who feel a new sensation with an implant quickly adapt and soon do not even notice it.

One of the advantages to implants is that as your face subtly continues to change with time, you have the option of later adding other types of tissue augmentation over them, such as autologous fat, to maintain the firm, youthful contours.

Potential Risks

An allergic response to either bovine or donor collagen (derived from tissue banks) is possible, although allergy testing should forestall this problem. Tissue rejection is possible with some of the biological filler products; however, it is a rare occurrence.

Now and then, filler treatments may produce a "lumpy" appearance in the skin.

As autologous fat is reabsorbed by the body, it can sometimes happen in an irregular way, creating an uneven surface. Also, there is some risk of infection at the site where fat is harvested and at the injection site.

There is a small risk of inflammation or infection at the ends of thread-like implants where they meet the suture areas; prophylactic (preventative) antibiotics may be prescribed to prevent this. Sometimes, an implant may later appear to have moved or shifted. If you sense this, see your doctor, who can remove and reinsert it.

Questions to Ask Your Doctor

- What type of filler treatment is appropriate for me?
- Do I need an allergy skin test?
- What kind of pain medication is available to me?
- How quickly will I recover?

- Can you show me before-and-after photos of other patients?
- How should I care for my skin before and after the filler?
- Should I stop taking my usual medications or supplements?

Eight
Lip Augmentation

Lip Augmentation

*Y*our genes may have granted you a beautiful Cupid's bow, but time and nature may have dimmed the dazzle of your smile. As we age, tissues in the lips begin to thin, and the lips may appear flatter and narrower. Sometimes the upper lip will sag, or an asymmetry in the shape of the lips will become more pronounced.

These changes can be disconcerting, particularly for women whose favorite makeup ritual is applying lipstick. As lips lose their natural contours, lips' edges sometimes lose definition too, so color is harder to apply and may smear or "bleed" into the surrounding areas. And if you've been a smoker, from all that pursing and puffing you may have developed wrinkles not only on the upper lip but also on the lips' surface.

Fortunately, modern lip augmentation procedures can reverse these changes and enhance the shape and fullness of your lips. Materials used to plump or reshape the lips are derived from a variety of substances, both biological and synthetic. Determining the specific materials to be used for your procedure and whether you will receive injections or solid implants will depend on the shape and condition of your lips and the results you seek.

Your doctor can help you decide which procedure will provide the best solution for you.

What Lip Augmentation Does

Lip fillers create instantaneous volume in one or both of the lips. The change can be dramatic, giving you a fuller, younger-looking mouth. Through injection or implant, lip augmentation enlarges or "fattens" the outer portion of the lips, called the *vermilion*. Augmentation softens fine lines within the lips and can reshape the Cupid's bow or better define your lips' edges.

Lip Augmentation with Injections

Most injectable lip treatments are temporary because the material is eventually reabsorbed by the body. Treatments are quick and easy to repeat, so people who are pleased with the results often choose to continue them. Temporary injectables include collagen and fat or fascia (derived from your own or donor tissue).

Longer-lasting treatments, considered semipermanent, involve the injections of the hybrids, material discussed in chapter 6. The hybrids contain microscopically tiny plastic spheres, blended in liquid collagen, which stimulates the growth of your own collagen. The result is fuller lips.

A permanent injection material, silicone in micro-droplet injection form, is used by some physicians who believe that, used appropriately, it is safe and effective. But many doctors avoid silicone because of its history of shifting or hardening in some patients.

Lip Augmentation with Implants

Lip augmentation with implants is semi-permanent or permanent. Two types of implants are available for this procedure: injectable implants and solid implants. *Injectable implants* are those consisting of tiny synthetic particles suspended in an injection fluid. The particles themselves permanently expand lip tissue, and they also signal your body to grow new collagen around them, which enhances the lips' fullness. Another injectable, the *bio-implant*, contains treated donor tissue such as fat, fascia, or collagen. Your own collagen uses this material as a scaffold, gradually anchoring itself to the product in a way that produces long-lasting changes.

> *I had implants in both lips. The doctor threaded what looked like a string of marshmallow into my lips. I had a local anesthetic, so there was no pain. My lips were a little sore at the corners. The procedure really plumped up my lips. I'm very pleased.*
>
> Karen, 34

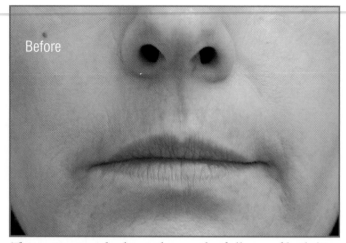

This patient wished to enhance the fullness of both lips.

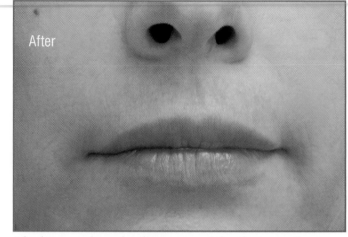

The human-based collagen, used for the procedure, will last for about six months.

Injectable solid implants are usually made of soft, moldable rubber. The material comes in narrow strips or porous tubes that are custom-trimmed for the desired lip shape. If for some reason you don't like the results, the implants can be removed or repositioned.

Are You a Candidate for Lip Augmentation?

Most people who want to have lip procedures done can tolerate the injections or implants very well. There are a few exceptions, however.

If you have a history of allergy to meat or other bovine products, or severe allergies in general, you may need to avoid bovine collagen. If you have any disorders involving collagen, raised scars, or connective tissue, such as *lupus* or *scleroderma*, these procedures may not be for you. Likewise, clotting disorders, poorly controlled diabetes, or allergies to local anesthetics may mean that you're not a good candidate for lip implants.

100

Finally, a history of cold sores or the oral herpes simplex virus may rule out lip augmentation. If the virus is present in your skin, it may be activated by the procedures. In many cases, antiviral medications can protect you from these complications. Your doctor will advise you.

Preparing for a Lip Augmentation Procedure

See your dentist beforehand if any dental work is needed, particularly for removal of excessive plaque. This plaque can increase the risk of infection. Your mouth is already a bacteria-rich environment, so preventing infection is particularly important for lip procedures.

If your treatment of choice is collagen injection, your doctor will give you a simple skin allergy test several weeks beforehand. You'll want to watch the injection test site, the inside of the forearm, closely for signs of bovine allergy. Symptoms of allergic reactions include a raised red lump that may itch, rash, hives, joint and muscle pain, headache, and in

Lip Augmentation Materials

Lip Implants	Injectables
Gore-Tex	Bovine collagen
Softform	Isolagen
UltraSoft	Restylane
Alloderm	Hylaform
Advanta	Artecoll
Dermis grafts	Argiform
Tendon grafts	Perlane
	Radiance
	CosmoDerm

a few cases, severe reactions that include shock and difficulty breathing.

Before an implant procedure, your doctor may advise you to stop taking certain medications. Taking aspirin and other blood-thinning drugs or herbal supplements is generally not advisable before any procedure requiring an incision. The doctor's decision to suspend the use of specific medication will depend on your individual health history. And of course, stop smoking! It slows healing and new tissue growth, and the pursing and puffing can create new lip wrinkles or may even distort the treatment results.

If you're going to be sedated before an implant procedure or twilight anesthesia will be used, your doctor will advise you to arrange for someone to drive you to and from the procedure and help you out at home until all traces of wooziness are gone.

How Are Lip Augmentation Injections Performed?

Most lip augmentation injections involve a very simple process and little or no discomfort. Done in the doctor's office, the procedure will require that you be draped as you lie on a table. Your doctor will numb your lips with a local anesthetic such as lidocaine placed on cotton swabs and then do a nerve block. You may want to ask if you can take a muscle relaxant or another mild sedative before you start. It usually takes a series of twelve to sixteen injections to complete the job. On the upside, the procedure won't take long, usually not more than twenty to thirty minutes. Your lips will stay numb for about an hour.

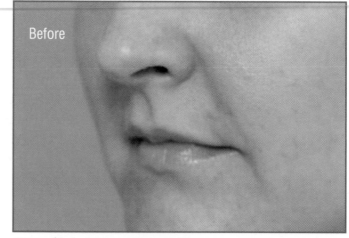

Upper lip prior to augmentation.

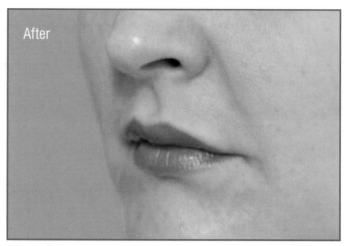

Upper lip augmentation with a permanent implant.

If you are having fat from your own body transferred to your lips, it's a little more complicated than a simple injection, because the doctor will be using a narrow tool, a *canula*, to create a tubular hollow inside your lips to receive the fat cells. For this you'll also be given a nerve-block anesthetic, which will numb your lips completely. This is a deeper injection of anesthetic into the lip sensory nerve.

Once the fat has been removed with a syringe from another part of your body, such as the abdomen, it's spun in a *centrifuge* to separate the fat from other fluids. Then, your doctor loads the liquid fat into a syringe and injects it into your lips.

How Is Lip Augmentation with Implants Performed?

First, the lips are disinfected and a local anesthetic is injected. Next, implants require that four tiny incisions be made, one at the very outer corner of each lip. (These well-hidden locations result in no visible scarring, however.)

With a special threading device, the implant material is pulled from one tiny incision at the corner of each lip through the lip to the other corner. Next, the ends are trimmed and rounded and single, hair-thin stitches are placed using dissolving or non-dissolving suture material. If your doctor prefers to use sutures that need to be removed, he or she will do so at a follow-up appointment in seven to ten days.

The extra swelling naturally resulting from an implant procedure will cause some pressure and discomfort; however, the residual numbness in your lips will last for several days and lessen any lingering discomfort. After the preliminary swelling subsides, you can take pain medication prescribed by your doctor if you feel you need it.

> *I wanted to get rid of creases around the borders of my lips, where my lipstick was bleeding. I had my lips injected with a semi-permanent filler. It worked wonderfully.*
>
> Kristen, 38

How Will I Look?

Lip augmentation produces an instant change in your appearance. You'll leave the doctor's office or clinic with fuller, curvier lips. Don't expect the Hollywood "bee-stung" lips sported by many actresses and models, however, unless that was the effect you asked your doctor to achieve. In most cases, lip augmentation produces results that are quite natural-looking.

If you've had lip augmentation through injection, you'll have some swelling immediately after the treatment, so expect some reduction in fullness over the next week before your lips settle into their new shape.

> *I am thrilled with my lip implants, and they do not affect the way my lips feel. When my husband kisses me, I can't even tell I have the implants. There is no change in sensation.*
>
> Jennifer, 28

After a solid implant or fat transfer procedure, you'll have more swelling initially, but the extra fullness will subside during the first week. You may also have temporary bruising on your lips, and once the anesthetic wears off, they will be very sensitive to pressure for a week or so.

Follow-Up Care

After most injections, patients receive a prescription for antibiotics to help avoid infection. To help reduce swelling during the first couple of days, you can apply an ice pack for fifteen minutes every hour or two.

Your lips are likely to feel numb after receiving implants, so be aware that eating may be awkward at first. You may want to stock up on liquid protein drinks and sip your meals through a straw for a few days. Soft foods like applesauce, pudding, or well-cooked vegetables will soon be easy to handle, and after about a week, you should be eating normally.

For fat injections or implant procedures, it will be important to avoid moving or stretching your mouth a great deal for about a week. Grimacing, huge yawns, big laughs, and the like may "shift" the implant material before it has become firmly anchored in place. (If you feel that any sort of shift has taken place, see your doctor.) Your doctor will explain exactly what degree of caution is necessary for the particular procedure you've chosen.

Your doctor may advise you to avoid lipstick for a few days, but that's only to avoid

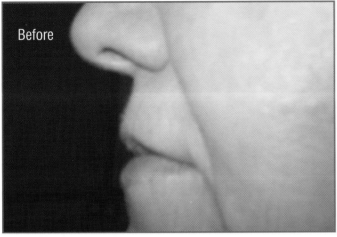

Upper lip before augmentation with an injectable soft-tissue filler.

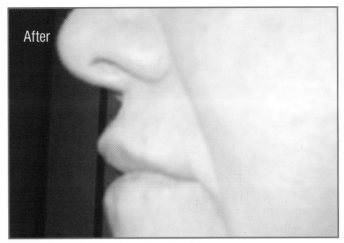

Upper lip after injections of a filler.

the pressure of its application. If you prefer to apply lip color right away, ask your doctor what kinds are appropriate. Some liquid lipsticks that are applied with a soft brush may be fine.

How Long Will Results Last?

Although it varies from person to person, temporary injectable lip treatments, such as those with collagen, usually last for about three to four months. Hyaluronic acid in the lips lasts eight to nine months. As the material is reabsorbed by your body, you'll notice a gradual reduction in lip fullness. You can decide whether you'd like to repeat the treatments.

Solid implants produce permanent lip changes, so there is no need to repeat these procedures unless for some reason you are not happy with the results and want the implants removed. (In rare cases, people find it difficult to adjust to the feel of an implant, or may feel conscious of it while kissing, for example.)

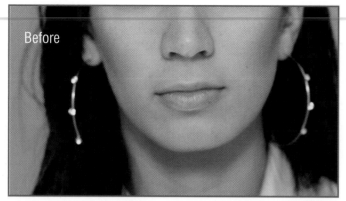

This woman wanted her upper lip to match the natural fullness of her lower lip.

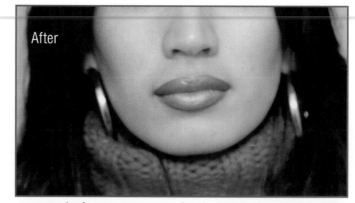

A strand of permanent implant material was inserted into her upper lip.

Although micro- and bio-implants are not removable, bio-implants will be absorbed by the patient over time.

As years pass, a small degree of shrinkage of the surface lip tissue still will occur. However, with permanent implants in place, shrinkage will be far less than normal.

Potential Risks

An allergic response to either bovine or donor collagen (derived from tissue banks) is possible, although allergy testing should forestall this problem. Very rarely, tissue rejection is a possibility with some of the biological filler injections.

On occasion, augmentation treatments may produce "lumpy" lips. As injected fat is reabsorbed by the body, it can sometimes create an uneven surface. Also, there is some risk of infection at the site where fat is harvested and at the injection sites.

There is a risk of inflammation or infection at the ends of lip implants where they meet the suture area, but careful trimming and rounding of the implant ends during the procedure should prevent irritation within the lip tissue that can cause this. Prophylactic (preventative) antibiotics may be prescribed for extra insurance against infection. More rarely, an implant may later appear to have moved or shifted. In that case, removal and retreatment may be required.

Questions to Ask Your Doctor

- What type of lip augmentation is appropriate for me?

- Do I need an allergy skin test?

- What kind of pain medication will be available to me?

- How quickly will I recover?

- If I've chosen temporary injections, how often will I need to repeat them?

- Can you show me before-and-after photos of other patients?

- How should I care for my lips before and after my treatment?

- Should I stop taking my usual medications or supplements?

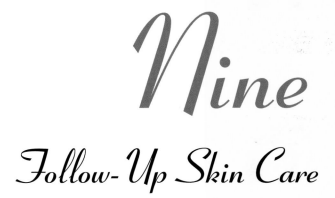

Nine

Follow-Up Skin Care

Follow-Up Skin Care

You've invested time and money to rejuvenate your skin—and it was worth it. Your skin looks younger and smoother, and you feel great about that. Now comes the crucial question. How do you keep your new glow?

We'll sum up your most important strategy in three words: avoid the sun. You can't do that completely, of course, unless you live in a cave. But sun damage is skin's Enemy Number One, and your renewed skin surface is especially vulnerable. So let's look at the best ways to protect your skin from those damaging rays, and consider often-overlooked healthy skin habits that can make a big difference in keeping your skin looking nearly as youthful as you feel.

Sun Protection Tips

Whether your skin is fair, olive-toned, or dark, the sun ages it. The damage is just less visible in people who naturally have more dark pigment. If your skin is tanning, it's taking a beating.

- *Try to stay indoors during the hours when the sun is strongest.* This is usually from 10:00 A.M. to 3:00 P.M. That's when ultraviolet rays are shortest and reach the earth's surface—and your skin's surface—most directly, delivering a powerful radiation punch.

- *Dress to protect your skin when outdoors.* Ever notice that people in very hot climates don't go bare-skinned? Even in desert heat, they wear long, flowing clothes. Fortunately, you don't have to be a nomad to dress for the sun—several smart manufacturers have developed lightweight clothing with a special weave that protects you just like sunscreen.

- *Don't forget a broad-brimmed hat.* That extra shade helps protect your face from radiation. A baseball cap's okay, but a minimum four-inch brim all the way around is even better. That also offers some coverage for your neck and shoulders.

- *Wear sunglasses.* They shield not only your eyes, but also the skin around them. The best are wraparound styles that offer sidepiece protection all the way to your temples. (They'll also keep you from squinting, which encourages crow's feet.)

Sunscreen Secrets

Many people don't realize that radiation reaches right through windows and can even penetrate most clothing. The sun subtly, slowly ages your skin year-round. That's why you need to wear sunscreen all over, every day, no matter what the season. And there are plenty of

---

Sunglasses Tip

Make sure your sunglasses have 100% UV-A and UV-B protection. Wear them on overcast days, too. Even though clouds block solar brightness, 80% of UV light still reaches your eyes and skin.

---

ways to maximize the power of sunscreen to protect your skin.

- *Use enough sunscreen.* That's not a pea-sized spot or two. That means using a brimming shot glass—a full ounce is what it takes to protect your skin adequately. One good strategy is to find a brand with a scent and texture you like and simply use it as your allover moisturizer. And keep a spray sunscreen handy to use on your back.

- *Use the right kind of sunscreen.* SPF stands for Sun Protection Factor. The number indicates how much longer you can be in the sun without damage than if you weren't wearing the sunscreen. For example, if your unprotected skin usually starts to burn or tan in about ten minutes and you wear an SPF 15, you are normally protected for about 150 minutes, or fifteen times longer. Err on the side of caution, but generally, if you have medium or dark-toned skin, SPF 15 will do. If you're fair-skinned, choose SPF 30 or higher. (If you think clothing will protect your skin, note that T-shirt fabric offers you an SPF of only 3.)

- *Be sure your sunscreen is full-spectrum.* Look for one that says "UV-A/UV-B protection" on the label. This shields you not only from the UV-B rays that cause obvious burning or tanning, but also from the UV-A rays that penetrate more deeply into the skin, weakening collagen and contributing to wrinkling and other long-term signs of age.

- *Check the ingredients.* The best sunscreens include particles of *titanium dioxide*, ground so fine that they actually sit within pores and block the rays like tiny mirrors. *Zinc oxide* is also very effective, and the newer zinc oxide products are nearly transparent, unlike the pastes you've seen on lifeguards' noses. Effective chemical sunscreens include combinations of ingredients such as para-aminobenzoic acid (PABA), cinnamates, benzophenes, anthranilates, and Parasol 1789. Each of these blocks UV-B or UV-A rays at different strengths.

- *Wait a minimum of thirty minutes after applying sunscreen before you go outside.* It takes that long before it begins to work. Then, reapply several times during the day—more often if you're active outdoors or you've been perspiring or swimming.

More Sun Protection Tips

So you're under a palm tree, sipping a drink with an umbrella in it. Better yet, you're under the umbrella, leaving the beach to people who want to wind up looking like old leather. Good move! But are you really out of the weather, skin-wise?

Not necessarily. Reflected sunlight, bouncing off any light-colored surface such as sand, snow, water, or even a sidewalk, also does real damage to your skin. That's why although staying out of direct sunlight helps, you still

History of the Sun Tan

Tanning first became popular in the 1920s when designer Coco Chanel returned with tanned skin after a cruise on a friend's yacht. Before then, women went to great lengths to keep their skin as white as possible. Tans were a sign of outdoor labor and lower-class status.

need to wear sunscreen. An amazing amount of radiation can sneak into what looks like shade.

Mourning the golden tan you used to think looked so healthy? You can enjoy a fashionable tan—as long as it's fake. Today's self-tanners won't turn you orange as the older ones did; you can get a very natural-looking glow. Try a few different products to see which looks best on you. Once you find one you like, mix it with a little moisturizer to help it go on more smoothly. Go lightly on rougher areas such as elbows and knees, which can soak up too much color, and wash your hands thoroughly right after you apply.

Most important, remember that the color gives you no sun protection whatsoever, so always top it off with sunscreen. You might want to apply a self-tanner before bed, then your sunscreen in the morning.

Healthy Skin Habits

Sun protection takes care of your skin from the outside in. But there are also major ways you can guard your skin that work from the inside out.

Don't Smoke

You've read how drawing on a cigarette contributes to those little vertical lip lines, and that squinting against smoke causes crow's feet. Smoking also damages your skin from the inside. Nicotine constricts blood flow, preventing fresh oxygen and nutrients from nourishing your skin. Starved for breath, your skin turns pasty and sallow and is much slower to heal from any irritation or wound. So let your skin breathe, and along with the rest of you, it will heal.

If you've struggled to quit before, don't give up. One of the most encouraging facts about ex-smokers is that most people who finally quit for good did so only after repeated attempts. So take a new attitude: you haven't failed, you're closer to success. Get help from your doctor, or the American Cancer Society, or join a class. There are many new ways to quit today. You'll live longer and look younger while you do!

Choose a Healthful Diet

The diet that's good for your skin is good for the rest of you too. To keep your skin looking youthful, feed it right. Your skin is your body's largest organ, and it responds wonderfully to nourishing food.

> *Equally important to the successful outcome of cosmetic procedures are realistic expectations on the part of the patient as well as the surgeon.*
> William Truswell, M.D.
> Facial Plastic Surgeon

If you've been haphazard about nutrition, educate yourself. There are hundreds of good books on healthful eating. Avoid the fads, and aim for a well-balanced diet that includes plenty of fruits, vegetables, whole grains, and lean protein. Junk foods that are fatty, processed, and full of artificial ingredients can make your skin look junky, too.

It's best to rely on wholesome food for most of your nutrients, but don't forget a multi-vitamin, calcium, and other supplements your doctor recommends. There's no need for fistfuls of pills, but you might ask a nutritionist how to get extra *antioxidants* into your diet. These powerhouse substances fight destructive molecules called *free radicals*, which do tremendous damage to body tissues, including your skin. Vitamins C and E are among the major antioxidants, and the skin-nourishing potential of these and other nutrients is being constantly studied. (You'll also see many new lotions with added antioxidants. Vitamin C serums can help to guard the skin from sun damage, but these products are fragile and don't keep their effectiveness long. And despite its importance in your diet, there's no reliable evidence that topical vitamin E does anything for your skin.)

Your skin's thirsty, too. Drink five to eight glasses of water every day. Dehydration dries out skin. (Afterall, it's 80 percent water!) A steady supply helps plump skin cells and keeps them looking healthier.

Watch out for alcohol, though. Moderate drinking is all your skin can tolerate and stay looking good. Excessive alcohol dilates blood vessels, weakens cell walls, and over time contributes to a bloated, sallow complexion. To spare your liver and your skin, drink only in moderation. Most medical sources define that as no more than one drink a day.

Smart Skin Care

The real secret about good skin care? It's not complicated. You just need to understand a few basics, learn what's good for your individual needs, and keep it simple. Choose cleansing products according to your skin type. There are four main skin types, and one easy way to find out your own: take the "tissue test." Wash your face clean, wait fifteen minutes, and then press a tissue over your skin.

Oily Skin

If the tissue is covered with shiny spots, your skin is oily. Your oil glands work overtime, giving you a steady sheen. You may also have visible pores.

Here's the best daily routine for oily skin. Wash your face morning and night with a cleanser that contains an alpha hydroxy acid, or AHA. Use an oil-free sun block in the morning and an oil-free moisturizer at night. If you wear makeup, use oil-free foundation, but sparingly. If you're still too shiny, try an over-the-counter low-strength peroxide or vitamin A solution after cleansing.

Combination Skin

If there's oil on the tissue but it seems to come mainly from the nose and forehead area, the "T-zone," you have combination skin (your cheeks are more dry).

Your oily areas may be a by-product of *seborrhea*, a condition that causes glands in the scalp and face to go into overdrive. Ask your doctor if that's the case, and if so, use an antiseborrheic shampoo and avoid hairstyling products that can creep onto the forehead, clogging pores.

Use a gentle, soapless cleanser for daily washing, and oil-free sunblocks and nighttime moisturizers. To soothe your dry areas, use a moisturizing mask on cheeks and neck only, once or twice a week.

Dry Skin

If the tissue shows no traces of oil, your skin is dry. You'll know this without the tissue test, however, because of the tight feeling and mild flakiness. Your main task with dry skin is simply to keep it well hydrated and use plenty of rich moisturizers.

For cleansing, use a liquid soapless cleanser. The most important tip is to then apply your moisturizing lotion or cream while your skin is still damp. It may not absorb immediately, but when it does, it will help "lock" the water's moisture into your skin.

After moisturizer, apply an oil-based sunscreen. Use a rich, hydrating moisturizer at night, and treat yourself to a weekly moisturizing mask. And drink plenty of water, to help replenish your skin from within.

> *Patient aftercare is very important. A plastic surgeon should be experienced so he or she can identify any problem quickly and resolve it.*
>
> Michael Byun, M.D.
> Plastic Surgeon

Normal Skin

If the tissue shows little to no oil, you're in luck—your skin's normal. This gives you a wider choice of products and cleansing routines.

Even so, never skip your sunblock, of course. For cleansing, use whatever product leaves your skin feeling comfortably supple.

Don't avoid moisturizers, but for routine use, oil-free brands will probably suit you best. When you feel your skin edging toward dryness, such as during the winter months, switch to something creamier for a while.

Prescription Products

Your skin may have special needs that over-the-counter brands don't adequately address, or you may simply want the most potent anti-aging products available. Your doctor can prescribe several for maintaining your skin in the best possible condition and slowing signs of age.

Tretinoin (Retin-A, Renova, Avita)

Originally prescribed to treat acne, Retin-A has since become a popular weapon against fine wrinkles and other signs of sun damage such as pigmented spots and rough patches. Along with smoothing the skin, Retin-A also produces a rosy glow. The active ingredient in Retin-A is *tretinoin*, a derivative of vitamin A.

Although most people can adapt to Retin-A if it's introduced gradually into the skin-care regimen, others find it too drying and irritating. New formulas, including Retin-A Micro, Renova, and Avita (available in cream or gel), allow your doctor to prescribe the version that's best for your skin.

Tretinoin products do increase your sun sensitivity, however, so if you begin using them, be even more vigilant about sun protection.

Bleaching Creams

If you're troubled by persistent or spreading age spots, a prescription cream containing hydroquinone can reduce or eliminate the extra-dark pigment. These creams are also effective against melasma, the darkened areas that can crop up on your skin during times of surging hormone production, such as pregnancy.

Like tretinoin products, bleaching creams increase dryness and make your skin much more vulnerable to the effects of the sun (which can cause *new* age spots), so using them will require extra vigilance in your sunscreen routines.

A Closing Note

You've learned about many techniques and healthy habits that can help you maintain your skin in the best possible condition for many years to come. Hopefully, you now have a much better idea about which of these treatments or procedures may be right for you.

What to expect from here? There will be many new developments in cosmetic treatments. Meanwhile, enjoy your newly rejuvenated skin. Care for it responsibly and let it joyfully express the "true you." You will always be just as young as you feel!

> *Proper skin care is important to maintaining the results of any facial rejuvenation procedure.*
>
> Jon Mendelsohn, M.D.
> Facial Plastic Surgeon

Resources

American Academy of Facial Plastic and Reconstructive Surgery

310 South Henry Street
Alexandria, VA 22314
Phone: 703-299-9291
Fax: 703-299-8898
www.facial-plastic-surgery.org

The American Academy of Facial Plastic and Reconstructive Surgery represents more than 2,700 facial plastic and reconstructive surgeons throughout the world. The AAFPRS is a National Medical Specialty Society of the American Medical Association. AAFPRS members are board-certified surgeons whose focus is surgery of the face, head, and neck.

The Web site offers a "virtual exam"—an interactive feature that highlights the most common areas in which facial cosmetic procedures are performed. The online Patient Information Series explains procedures, helps you determine whether they're right for you, and lets you know what to expect. Also on the site are FAQs, before-and-after photos, a physician finder, and a quarterly online magazine.

The American Society for Aesthetic Plastic Surgery

11081 Winners Circle
Los Alamitos, CA 90720
Phone: 800-364-2147 or 562-799-2356
Fax: 562-799-1098
www.surgery.org

Founded in 1967, ASAPS is a professional organization of plastic surgeons, certified by the American Board of Plastic Surgery, who specialize in cosmetic plastic surgery. The organization has 1,900 members in the U.S. and Canada, as well as corresponding members in many other countries. The Web site can help you find a surgeon and offers an "Ask an ASAPS Surgeon" feature, as well as news, updates, and consumer-oriented reports on surgical and nonsurgical procedures. The site also has a Find-a-Surgeon feature. You'll also find numerous articles and procedure descriptions, some in both English and Spanish.

American Society of Plastic Surgeons

444 East Algonquin Road
Arlington Heights, IL 60005
Phone: 847-228-9900
www.plasticsurgery.org

The American Society of Plastic Surgeons is the largest plastic-surgery specialty organization in the world. Founded in 1931, the society is composed of board-certified plastic surgeons who perform cosmetic and reconstructive surgery.

The mission of ASPS is to advance quality care to plastic surgery patients by encouraging high standards of training, ethics, physician practice and research in plastic surgery. The society advocates for patient safety, such as encouraging its members to operate in surgical facilities that have passed rigorous external review of equipment and staffing. The society works in concert with the Plastic Surgery Educational Foundation, founded in 1948, which supports research and educational programs for plastic surgeons.

On the society's Web site are FAQs, a history of plastic surgery, a surgeon finder, capsule descriptions of procedures, patient profiles, a photo gallery, and cost information.

American Board of Plastic Surgery

Seven Penn Center
Suite 400
1635 Market Street
Philadelphia, PA 19103-2204
Phone: 215-587-9322
Fax: 215-587-9622
www.abplsurg.org

The mission of The American Board of Plastic Surgery is to promote safe, ethical, efficacious plastic surgery to the public by maintaining high standards for the education, examination, and certification of plastic surgeons as specialists and subspecialists. Primarily for physicians, the board's Web site includes FAQs explaining how doctors become board-certified and describing differences among licensure, certification, and accreditation.

American Academy of Cosmetic Surgery

Cosmetic Surgery Information Service
737 North Michigan Avenue
Suite 820
Chicago, IL 60611
Phone: 312-981-6760
www.cosmeticsurgery.org

Formed in 1985, the American Academy of Cosmetic Surgery represents practitioners of medical disciplines including dermatology, ophthalmology, otorhinolaryngology, plastic and reconstructive surgery, oral and maxillofacial surgery, general surgery, and others. The AACS is the nation's largest organization representing cosmetic surgeons.

The Academy's purpose is to maintain a membership of medical and dental professionals who participate in postgraduate medical education opportunities, specifically in cosmetic surgery, so that the public is assured of receiving consistently high-quality medical and dental care.

The Academy's Web site offers assistance choosing and finding a surgeon, describes procedures and their risks, explains what to do before surgery, and helps you determine whether you're a good candidate.

American Society for Laser Medicine and Surgery

2404 Stewart Avenue
Wausau, WI 54401
Phone: 715-845-9283
Fax: 715-848-2493
E-mail: information@aslms.org
www.aslms.org

Founded in 1981 to educate both physicians and the lay public, the society maintains a

Web site with public-health information that includes an introduction to and history of lasers, online referral service, standards of practice, FAQs, and links to member Web sites.

American Academy of Dermatology

930 East Woodfield Road
Schaumburg, IL 60173
Phone: 847-330-0230
Fax: 847-330-0050
www.aad.org

The American Academy of Dermatology is the nation's largest dermatologic association. With a membership of more than 13,700, it represents virtually all practicing dermatologists in the United States. Public information on the Web site includes current and archived issues of the AAD's consumer magazine *Dermatology Insights;* free online "pamphlets" on surgical and nonsurgical cosmetic procedures; and help finding a dermatologist.

AAD operates another site, AgingSkinNet, at www.skincarephysicians.com, which offers descriptions and FAQs on medical and

surgical skin rejuvenation, chemical peeling, soft-tissue augmentation, botulinum toxin, dermabrasion, laser skin resurfacing, nonablative skin treatment, acne scar removal, hair removal, and more.

American Society for Dermatologic Surgery

5550 Meadowbrook Drive
Rolling Meadows, IL 60008
Phone: 847-956-0900
Consumer Hotline: 800-441-273
e-mail: info@aboutskinsurgery.com
www.aboutskinsurgery.com

The American Society for Dermatologic Surgery (ASDS) was founded in 1970 to promote excellence in the subspecialty of dermatologic surgery and to foster high standards of patient care. The society's Web site offers information about dermatologic-surgery practice, tips on choosing the right surgeon, a surgeon-search link, charts and descriptions of common skin conditions and treatments, and before-and-after photos.

American Skin Association, Inc.

346 Park Avenue South, 4th Floor
New York, NY 10010
Phone: 800-499-SKIN or 212-889-4858
Fax: 212-889-4959
E-mail: info@skinassn.org
www.skinassn.org

The American Skin Association is a patient-advocacy group that supports research and education on skin disorders. For a membership fee of $25.00, you'll receive the quarterly newsletter *SKINFacts,* educational brochures on specific skin disorders, and notices of public forums and meetings.

The U.S. National Library of Medicine

8600 Rockville Pike
Bethesda, MD 20894
www.nlm.nih.gov
www.nlm.nih.gov/medlineplus

The National Library of Medicine Web site indexes articles from more than 3,500 medical journals. The service is aimed primarily at scientists and health professionals; however MEDLINEplus is written for consumers.

eMedicine, Inc.

1004 Farnam Street, Suite 300
Omaha, Nebraska 68102
Phone: 402-341-3222
Fax: 402-341-3336
www.emedicine.com

Though created for an audience of health professionals, the eMedicine Web site includes informative descriptions of hundreds of procedures. Launched in 1996, the site is the most comprehensive source of information available free online about procedures, risks, side effects, anesthesia, preparation for surgery, follow-up, expectations, and other pertinent information. Nearly 10,000 physician authors and editors contribute to the eMedicine Clinical Knowledge Base.

The American Board of Facial Plastic and Reconstructive Surgery

115C South St. Asaph Street
Alexandria, Virginia 22314
Phone: 703-549-3223
Fax: 703-549-3357
www.abfprs.org

This organization's mission is improving the quality of facial plastic surgery available to the public by measuring the qualifications of candidate surgeons against certain rigorous standards. To be considered for membership, a physician must have completed a residency program and have been in practice a minimum of two years, have one hundred operative reports accepted by a peer-review committee, successfully pass an 8-hour written and oral examination, and hold the appropriate licensure and adhere to the ABFPRS Code of Ethics.

American Board of Medical Specialties

1007 Church Street Suite 404
Evanston, IL 60201-5913
Phone: 847-491-9091
Fax: 847-328-3596
www.abms.org

The American Board of Medical Specialties is an organization of twenty-four approved medical specialty boards. The intent of the certification of physicians is to provide assurance to the public that those certified by an ABMS Member Board have successfully completed an approved training program and an evaluation process assessing their ability to provide quality patient care in the specialty. This Web site explains how specialists are trained and certified; it also offers a search feature for finding certified physicians.

123

Glossary

A

ablative laser: a laser capable of *ablating* (carrying away, removing) a layer of skin.

abrasion: the wearing away of a substance, such as skin; also a superficial injury to the skin (or other body tissue) caused by rubbing or scraping.

Accutane: a drug that treats acne by reducing the amount of oil produced by the skin's sebaceous (oil) glands.

acetylcholine: a naturally occurring chemical that carries information across the space between two nerve cells.

actinic keratosis: a flat, scaly skin lesion, usually slightly raised and red or pink in color, on a sun-exposed surface. About 20 percent of such lesions are precancerous.

aesthetic surgery: See *cosmetic surgery*.

aesthetician: a nonmedical practitioner who specializes in noninvasive skin treatments, such as facials, light chemical peels, exfoliation, and general skin care.

age spot: a flat patch of raised, brown pigmentation on the skin, often caused by sun exposure and more common with aging. Age spots are not considered medically dangerous.

AHA: See *alpha hydroxy acid*.

alexandrite laser: amplified light, used primarily for the treatment of hair or pigmented skin lesions, that removes both natural and unnatural pigmentation (such as a tattoo) from the skin.

alpha hydroxy acid: one of a group of naturally occurring acids, often derived from foods (such as fruits and milk) that remove layers of dead skin cells and encourage cell regeneration.

ambulatory care: medical care given on an outpatient basis.

aminoglycosides: a group of broad-spectrum antibiotics, such as streptomycin and neomycin, that reduce bacterial protein synthesis.

anesthetic: a drug that causes lack of sensation or unconsciousness. A *local anesthetic* targets a specific area of the body without putting the patient to sleep. A *general anesthetic* brings about unconsciousness.

anthranilate: a sun-blocking agent used in sunscreens.

anticoagulant: a substance that prevents blood clotting.

antioxidant: a synthetic or natural substance that reacts with oxygen to protect other compounds from oxygen's harmful effects. Vitamins A, C, and E, along with other nutrients, are antioxidants believed to prevent the damaging activity of free radicals in the body.

autologous fat: fatty tissue taken from one's own body to be used elsewhere on the body for contouring or filling.

B

benign growth: a noncancerous tumor or other swelling.

benzophenones: substances used in sunscreens and other products to prevent the breakdown of ingredients due to ultraviolet rays.

blood thinner: See *anticoagulant.*

blue peel: a chemical peel using trichloroacetic acid (TCA) and a blue dye, which improves the procedure's accuracy.

board-certified physician: a doctor who has completed a required course of study—including an accredited residency—in a medical specialty, and who has passed the certifying board's examination.

Botox: an injectable, medical-grade form of the botulinum toxin.

Botox injection: a medical procedure involving the injection of botulinum toxin for facial smoothing and contouring.

botulinum: a potent bacterial toxin produced by the organism *Clostridium botulinum.* Botulinum toxins are among the strongest poisons known, but the medical grade used in Botox is a weakened, nonlethal form.

botulism: a potentially deadly illness caused by one of the *Clostridium botulinum* toxins. There are four types of botulism infection: infant botulism, food-borne botulism, wound botulism, and botulism from an unknown source.

bovine collagen: collagen derived from cattle.

C

calcium channel blockers: drugs used to treat heart conditions (such as angina), hypertension, and stroke by inducing vascular and other smooth-muscle relaxation.

cannula: a hollow tube used in medical procedures, such as liposuction.

carbolic acid: See *phenol*.

carbon-dioxide laser: a device using high-energy light beams (continuous wave or pulsed) in which the primary medium is carbon-dioxide gas.

chemical peel: a facial-rejuvenation procedure using a chemical solution to peel away the outer layer or layers of skin. Most effective on fair, thin skin and superficial wrinkles, a chemical peel can reduce or eliminate fine lines, correct uneven pigmentation, remove keratoses and other skin growths, and minimize acne and related scarring.

cinnamates: sunscreen ingredients obtained from cinnamon oil, certain balsams, or storax. Cinnamates occasionally cause allergic reactions in some sunscreen users.

CO2 laser: See *carbon-dioxide laser*.

cold sore: a viral infection, caused by *Herpes simplex* type 1, of the lip or mouth. Cold sores can erupt as painful blisters, can be contagious, and can be controlled with antiviral medication. Illness, fever, stress, and sunlight can aggravate cold sores, which tend to be recurrent.

collagen injection: a cosmetic-surgery technique using collagen protein to correct wrinkles, scars, and skin depressions.

collagen: the major protein of scar tissue and skin, tendon, bone, cartilage, and other connective tissue. Collagen production is essential for healing.

cosmetic procedure: surgery—invasive or noninvasive—or other treatment to repair or reshape parts of the body, primarily to improve appearance rather than function.

cosmetology: the performance of nonmedical treatments—facials, exfoliation, masks, wraps, electrolysis, and "beauty treatments," for example—to improve appearance.

crow's feet: fine lines and wrinkles radiating from the eyes, caused by sun exposure, smiling, and squinting, and made worse by smoking.

D

deep peel: a surgical procedure using strong acids to dissolve outer skin layers and regenerate collagen in underlying skin.

dermabrasion: a surgical procedure that uses a high-speed rotating brush to remove the upper layers of skin in order to smooth away wrinkles, small scars, tattoos, and other facial flaws.

dermaplaning: a surgical procedure that uses a hand-held instrument called a dermatome to treat deep acne scars.

dermatologist: a medical doctor who specializes in treating skin disorders and defects.

dermis: the thickest of the skin layers, making up about 90 percent of the skin's thickness and containing protein fibers (collagen and elastin) that support lymph and blood vessels, nerves, muscle cells, sweat glands, sebaceous glands, and hair follicles.

diode laser: in cosmetic procedures, a device using high-intensity specialized light that passes through the skin to be selectively absorbed by blood vessels, causing them to disappear. The diode laser has a diode as its light source, as do familiar devices such as LED watches. Diode laser devices have different wavelengths for different applications. Commercially, they're used to read and burn CD's and DVD's. Cosmetically they are effective on spider veins, broken blood vessels, freckles, age spots, and rosacea pigmentation, and for hair removal.

donor tissue: fat or other substances taken from one person and injected or implanted into another during plastic-surgery and cosmetic procedures.

dynamic wrinkles: facial lines that appear and disappear with movement of the facial muscles.

E

EKG: See *electrocardiogram.*

elastin: a protein that gives the skin elasticity, tone, and texture.

electrocardiogram: a recording of the heart's electrical activity; used as a measure of heart health and strength.

epidermis: the skin's thin outer protective layer, which retains hydration and produces the pigment melanin. The topmost surface consists of dead skin cells, which are continually shed.

Erbium YAG laser: a device that produces high-intensity specialized light, though at a different wavelength than the CO laser. The latter is more effective in treating scars and wrinkles.

esthetic surgery: See *cosmetic procedure.*

esthetician: See *aesthetician.*

exfoliation: shedding or removal of cells from the skin or mucous membranes.

F

fascia lata: connective tissue surrounding the muscles of the thigh.

fat injection: placement of fatty tissue from one's own body or from a donor into another body site to smooth or augment parts of the body (usually the face or lips).

filler implant: a synthetic or organic material introduced into a face or other body part for smoothing, augmenting, or firming.

filler injection: a gel-like substance (often collagen) harvested from one's own or another's body and reintroduced, usually to smooth facial irregularities or wrinkles.

free radical: a chemically active atom or molecular fragment that contains too many or too few electrons and is therefore "charged." In the process of seeking or releasing electrons (within a human or other organism) to become stable, a free radical can damage body cells.

French peel: a term used variously to describe a form of microdermabrasion using aluminum-hydroxide pellets or a chemical peel using chlorophyll or lactic acids.

full-spectrum sunscreen: a product that protects skin from the sun, offering both UV-A and UV-B protection. In one study, a "full-spectrum" product formulated with Octocrylene and Parsol

1789 was more effective than a "broad-spectrum" product formulated with Octyl Methoxycinnamate and zinc oxide.

G

glabella: the space between the eyebrows.

glycolic acid: hydroxyacetic acid—often found in young plants and green fruits as a result of photosynthesis—used as an active agent in chemical peels.

H

hair follicle: in the epidermis, a tubelike opening where the hair shaft develops.

hemoglobin: the pigment that gives blood its characteristic red color; also the primary compound that combines with oxygen and carries it throughout the body.

herpes simplex virus: See *cold sore.*

hyaluronic acid: an acid which occurs naturally in our tissues and is also used commercially as an injectable implant to fill fine wrinkles and facial lines.

hydroquinone: a topical hypopigmenting agent that blocks the formation of pigments in the skin; used to diminish spots, freckles, melasma, and other hyperpigmented areas.

hyperpigmentation: excess skin pigmentation (coloring) as seen in age spots, freckles, port-wine birthmarks, and other comparatively dark spots or patches.

hypopigmentation: total or localized absence or deficiency of skin pigmentation (coloring).

I

implant: the invasive or noninvasive surgical introduction of an object or substance to improve the health or appearance of the body; used in facial cosmetic procedures to smooth and contour areas of the face.

incision: a cut made with a knife during a surgical procedure.

injectable implant: a substance that can be introduced into the body by injection rather than incision during plastic surgery or another cosmetic or surgical procedure.

intravenous: a method of administering fluids and/or medications through a vein.

invasive surgery: a surgical procedure that involves making an incision and exposing internal tissues or organs.

IV: See *intravenous.*

K

keloid: a raised scar, larger than the original wound, resulting from excessive collagen during connective-tissue healing. A keloid scar often itches, hurts, burns or continues to grow.

keratosis: a buildup of keratin—the hard protein in skin, nails, and hair—on the upper layer of skin. Common causes of keratosis are aging (senile keratosis) and sun exposure (actinic keratosis). Another form, keratosis pilaris, produces small rough bumps where keratin collects in hair follicles. See also *actinic keratosis.*

L

laser: acronym for Light Amplification by Stimulated Emission of Radiation; a specialized high-energy light beam.

laser skin resurfacing: smoothing the skin using laser-light beams to vaporize upper skin layers.

lidocaine: a local, nonsedating anesthetic used in some cosmetic and surgical procedures.

light peel: a chemical peel involving the skin's superficial layers and minimizing or removing skin "flaws" such as freckles, age spots, and fine lines and wrinkles.

lip augmentation: a cosmetic procedure that increases lip size and definition by injection of a soft-tissue filler, such as collagen, or by implanting synthetic or grafted material.

liposuction: removal of body fat using a suction device to improve the body's shape and contour.

local anesthetic: a nonsedating drug used to block pain sensations in a region of the body.

M

medium peel: a chemical peel that removes more skin layers than a light peel and is more effective in reducing the appearance of fine lines and wrinkles, acne and mild scarring, weathered skin, and hyperpigmentation. Light, medium, and deep peels are distinguished by the strength of the chemicals used.

melanin: a protective pigment contained in the skin and the eye to protect those organs from harmful sun radiation, through tanning, for example.

melanoma: a malignant (cancerous) tumor, arising from the melanocytic system of the skin and other organs.

melasma: a dark discoloration of the skin.

microdermabrasion: a cosmetic procedure, safer and less powerful than dermabrasion, that projects microcrystals onto the skin to remove outer cells and improve appearance.

micropigmentation: cosmetic tattooing to create a "permanent makeup" effect, usually on the lips, eyelids, and eyebrows.

myasthenia gravis: a rare, usually treatable, chronic neuromuscular disease that produces weakness and abnormally rapid fatigue of the voluntary muscles.

N

nasolabial crease: also called *nasolabial groove* or *nasolabial fold,* a furrow between the wing of the nose and the lip.

Nd:YAG laser: abbreviation for Neodymium:Yttrium Aluminum Garnet laser, which uses a synthetic crystal as the laser medium. (*Neodymium* is the rare earth element active in Nd:YAG and Md:Glass lasers.)

Neodymium laser: See *Nd:YAG laser.*

neurotransmitter: a chemical substance released by a transmitting neuron at the synapse that allows information to be transferred from one neuron to another.

nonablative laser: a skin-resurfacing device that passes through outer tissue (thus is nonexfoliating) and stimulates collagen creation in the dermis.

O

otolaryngologist: a physician who specializes in medical and surgical treatment of patients with conditions of the ear, nose, throat, and related structures of the head and neck.

P

PABA: P-aminobenzoic acid, which serves as an ultraviolet-light screen in lotions and creams.

penicillamine: a drug derived from penicillin used as antidote to some poisons and also used to treat rheumatoid arthritis.

Perlane: a product containing hyaluronic acid and used in cosmetic procedures to add volume to tissue, thus reshaping facial contours, correcting folds, or augmenting lips.

phenol: also called *carbolic acid,* a chemical used in deep peels to minimize sun damage and severe wrinkling.

photoaging: skin damage caused by the sun.

pigment: in humans, melanin and other types of coloring that give skin, blood, and other organic structures their tint.

plastic surgeon: a medical doctor who specializes in reducing scarring and disfigurement resulting from accidents, birth defects, and some diseases. A *cosmetic plastic surgeon* specializes in aesthetic improvement of the face and body via surgery. Plastic surgeons are cosmetic and reconstructive.

port wine stain: a flat type of hemangioma, a reddish-purple birthmark consisting of superficial blood vessels in the skin. These birthmarks can be raised and very large.

Power Peel: trademark technique of microdermabrasion in which microcrystals are projected onto the skin to remove dead skin cells. Cells and crystals are then vacuumed back into the microdermabrasion tool.

prophylactic: preventive; used to describe a treatment or medication.

psoriasis: a common chronic (though often sporadic) skin disorder involving scaly patches of various sizes and shapes.

pulsed dye laser: high-energy light using dye as a medium and delivered in pulses rather than continuous waves, used primarily on vascular lesions.

Q

quinine: an alkaloid used in the treatment of malaria and autoimmune disorders such as rheumatoid arthritis.

R

Renova: a brand name of the generic drug tretinoin, a medicine derived from vitamin A and used topically to reduce fine wrinkles and skin roughness and discoloration.

Restylane: an injectable gel that adds volume to the lips and lifts wrinkles and folds.

Retin-A: a brand name of the generic drug tretinoin, a medicine derived from vitamin A and used topically in the treatment of acne.

retinoid: a derivative of vitamin A used to treat skin conditions and for other medical applications.

rosacea: a common facial skin disorder involving chronic inflammation and redness of the cheeks, nose, chin, forehead, or eyelids. In advanced cases in men, the oil glands enlarge causing bulbous red swelling of the nose and cheeks.

ruby laser: light amplification produced by a crystal of sapphire (aluminum oxide) containing trace amounts of chromium oxide.

S

scleroderma: hardening of skin. Systemic scleroderma is an autoimmune disorder in which the immune system attacks the skin and potentially the lungs, esophagus, kidneys, and heart.

seborrhea: a skin disorder caused by excessive secretion of sebum—fat and cellular debris—from the sebaceous glands.

sedation: calming or rendering a patient unconscious with a sedative, a medication that promotes tranquility and sometimes sleep.

silicon: a nonmetallic mineral, the second-most-abundant element of the earth's crust (after oxygen).

skin resurfacing: removal of the outer layer or layers of the skin using abrasion, chemicals, or a laser.

solar elastosis: photodamage, usually in light-skinned people, characterized by massive deposits of thickened, tangled, and degraded collagen fibers damaged by exposure to intense sunlight and appearing as loose, sagging, tough skin.

SPF: See *sun-protection factor.*

spider veins: small clusters of red, blue, or purple veins, most often occurring on the thighs, calves, ankles, and just as often on the face.

static wrinkles: facial lines that appear independently of the movement of facial muscles.

stratum corneum epidermis: the outer layer of the epidermis, consisting of dead cells and acting as a barrier between the body and the environment.

subcutaneous: under the epidermis and dermis.

subcutis: also called *superficial fascia,* a loose, meshy layer beneath the skin containing fat, cutaneous vessels, and nerves.

sunblock: a lotion, cream, or gel used topically to prevent ultraviolet rays from penetrating the skin. The term is often used interchangeably with *sunscreen,* though a *sunblock* may contain opaque substances, such as zinc oxide, not necessarily present in sunscreen.

sun-protection factor: describing a sunscreen or sunblock, the number of hours the wearer could theoretically remain in the sun while absorbing an hour's worth of ultraviolet light. An SPF of 15 to 30 is usually recommended.

sunscreen: a liquid, lotion, cream, or gel used to prevent sun damage to the skin or hair. See also *sunblock* and *sun-protection factor.*

suture: a "stitch" made in the skin, usually with a synthetic thread (such as nylon), to close a wound. Some sutures are absorbable—they dissolve over time and don't require removal.

T

TCA: See *trichloroacetic acid.*

titanium dioxide: a substance used in some sunscreens and other creams and powders to protect the skin from external irritants, including the sun.

topical anesthetic: a local anesthetic applied externally as a liquid, cream, ointment, or gel.

tretinoin: an acid derived from vitamin A used in the treatment of skin disorders and irregularities such as acne, psoriasis, and fine wrinkles. Sold by prescription as Retin-A and Renova.

trichloroacetic acid: a chemical used in facial and other peels—light, medium, or heavy, depending on concentration and method of application.

twilight anesthetic: an intravenous sedative that induces relaxation but not unconsciousness (though some patients given a twilight anesthetic do fall asleep).

U

ultraviolet rays: electromagnetic radiation with wavelengths between X rays and visible light. UV-A, UV-B, and UV-C rays are ultraviolet rays distinguished by wavelength.

V

varicose veins: twisted, swollen blood vessels, often present in women's legs after one or more pregnancies, caused by weakening of the vascular walls.

Index

About the Authors

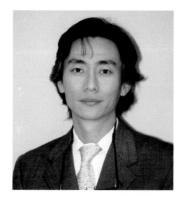

Michael Byun, M.D., is a plastic surgeon in private practice in Chicago, where he founded Chicago Cosmetic Surgery. Born in Tokyo, raised and educated in California, Dr. Byun graduated from the University of California, Irvine with high honors. He then attended Northwestern Medical School in Chicago and completed a clinical fellowship in Plastic Surgery at Northwestern. He served as research advisor at the University of California, Department of Neurobiology and at the National Institute of Neurological Disorders and Stroke Research.

Dr. Byun is board-certified by the American Board of Plastic Surgery. He is also a member of the American Medical Association, and a member of the American Society of Plastic Surgery. Dr. Byun is certified in Ultra Pulse Laser Resurfacing, Endoscopic Surgery in Plastic Surgery, Maxillofacial Principle and Technique, and Erbium Laser. He is recognized nationally as a mid-facelift surgeon, and has presented his work at conferences of the American Society of Aesthetic Plastic Surgery and American Society of Plastic Surgery.

Dr. Byun is an assistant professor at Rush University and the director of pediatric plastic surgery at Lutheran General Hospital. He has published numerous articles and has been a presenter at national and international plastic surgery conferences. He has been featured on FOX News and NBC News for his innovative procedures with Dermal Spin, a lip augmentation procedure, and the permanent wrinkle filler, *Radiance*.

Dr. Byun may be reached through his web site: Chicagocosmeticsurgery.com.

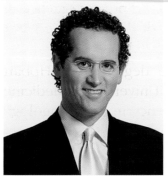

Jon Mendelsohn, M.D., is a facial plastic surgeon, and is the medical director of the Advanced Cosmetic Surgery & Laser Center, Cincinnati, Ohio. Dr. Mendelsohn received a bachelor of science degree in molecular biology from Syracuse University. He attended medical school at the State University of New York Health Science Center, Syracuse, and also completed a residency there in otolaryngology: head and neck surgery.

Dr. Mendelsohn is board-certified by the American Board of Facial Plastic and Reconstructive Surgery and the American Board of Otolaryngology—Head and Neck Surgery. He is a fellow of: the American Academy of Facial Plastic and Reconstructive Surgery, American College of Surgeons, American Academy of Facial Plastic and Reconstructive Surgery, and the American Academy of Otolaryngology—Head and Neck Surgery.

Dr. Mendelsohn is a member of the American Academy of Facial Plastic and Reconstructive Surgery's committees on multimedia and new technologies and devices. He is a national trainer in the use of Botox and a regional trainer in the use of autologous platlet gels. He has presented nationally at conferences on facial plastic surgery, and has authored numerous papers and publications on the topic of facial plastic surgery. Dr. Mendelsohn has also been awarded the Keeping America Strong Award; the national program, *Heartbeat of America*, hosted by William Shatner, salutes Dr. Mendelsohn's practice as a distinguished provider of plastic surgery.

Dr. Mendelsohn may be reached through his Website, www.351face.com, where he will feature updates on cosmetic procedures described in this book.

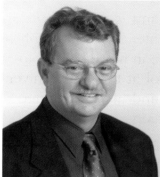

William H. Truswell, M.D., is a facial plastic surgeon in private practice in Northampton, Massachusetts. He is medical director of the Aesthetic Laser and Cosmetic Surgery Center, which he founded in 1976.

Dr. Truswell received a bachelor of science degree from Hobart College, Geneva, New York. He graduated from the University of Medicine and Dentistry of New Jersey, and completed a residency in otolaryngology and facial plastic and reconstructive surgery at the University of Connecticut School of Medicine.

Dr. Truswell is board-certified by the American Board of Facial Plastic and Reconstructive Surgery and the American Board of Otolaryngology. He is a fellow of the American College of Surgeons, the American Academy of Facial Plastic and Reconstructive Surgery, the American Academy of Cosmetic Surgery, the American Academy of Otolaryngology Head and Neck Surgery, and the American Society for Head and Neck Surgery.

Dr. Truswell is a clinical instructor in facial plastic surgery in the Division of Otolaryngology, Department of Surgery, University of Connecticut School of Medicine.

He is also a medical consultant to Atrium Medical Corporation Advanta for ePTFE facial soft tissue implants. He is the designer of the Truswell Insertion Instrument for soft-tissue implants, manufactured by Marina Medical Corporation.

A writer and lecturer, Dr. Truswell writes articles on facial plastic and reconstructive surgery in medical specialty journals, consults with other professionals for books on facial plastic surgery, and lectures at facial plastic surgery meetings throughout the country.

Dr. Truswell may be reached through his web site: www.truswellplasticsurg.com.

Consumer Health Titles from Addicus Books

Visit our online catalog at www.AddicusBooks.com

After Mastectomy—Healing Physically and Emotionally $14.95
Cancers of the Mouth and Throat—A Patient's Guide to Treatment $14.95
Cataracts: A Patient's Guide to Treatment $14.95
Colon & Rectal Cancer—A Patient's Guide to Treatment $14.95
Coping with Psoriasis—A Patient's Guide to Treatment $14.95
Coronary Heart Disease—A Guide to Diagnosis and Treatment $15.95
Countdown to Baby—The 100 Most Frequently Asked Questions by Expectant Mothers $14.95
Exercising Through Your Pregnancy $17.95
The Fertility Handbook—A Guide to Getting Pregnant $14.95
The Healing Touch—Keeping the Doctor/Patient Relationship Alive Under Managed Care $9.95
The Macular Degeneration Source Book $14.95
LASIK—A Guide to Laser Vision Correction $14.95
Living with P.C.O.S.—Polycystic Ovarian Syndrome $14.95
Lung Cancer—A Guide to Treatment & Diagnosis $14.95
The Macular Degeneration Source Book $14.95
The Non-Surgical Facelift Book —A Guide to Facial Rejuvenation Procedures $19.95
Overcoming Postpartum Depression and Anxiety $14.95
A Patient's Guide to Dental Implants $14.95
Prescription Drug Addiction—The Hidden Epidemic $15.95
Prostate Cancer—A Patient's Guide to Treatment $14.95
Simple Changes: The Boomer's Guide to a Healthier, Happier Life $9.95
A Simple Guide to Thyroid Disorders $14.95
Straight Talk About Breast Cancer —From Diagnosis to Recovery $14.95
The Stroke Recovery Book —A Guide for Patients and Families $14.95
The Surgery Handbook—A Guide to Understanding Your Operation $14.95
Understanding Lumpectomy—A Treatment Guide for Breast Cancer $14.95
Understanding Parkinson's Disease —A Self-Help Guide $14.95

Organizations, associations, corporations, hospitals, and other groups may qualify for special discounts when ordering more than 24 copies. For more information, please contact the Special Sales Department at Addicus Books. Phone (402) 330-7493.

Please send:

___copies of _____
                                             (Title of book)

at $_____each   TOTAL   _____

Nebr. residents add 5.5% sales tax   _____

Shipping/Handling
   $4.00 postage for first book.
   $1.00 for each additional book.   _____

TOTAL ENCLOSED: _____

Name _____

Address _____

City_____State_____Zip _____

          ☐   Visa   ☐   Master Card   ☐   Am. Express

Credit card number _____Expiration date _____

Order by credit card, personal check or money order. Send to:

Addicus Books
Mail Order Dept.
P.O. Box 45327
Omaha, NE 68145

Or, order TOLL FREE: **800-352-2873**

Online at: **www.AddicusBooks.com**